SPEED-STRENGTH TRAINING FOR FOOTBALL

Billy,

Keep it up!

K. Page

Holidays 2000

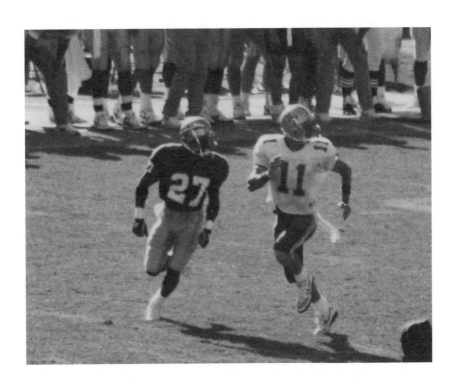

SPEED-STRENGTH TRAINING FOR FOOTBALL

by

E. J. "Doc" Kreis, DA
Middle Tennessee State University

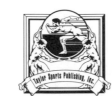

Taylor Sports Publishing, Inc.
Nashville, Tennessee

ISBN Number 0-9632677-0-1.

Copyright © 1992 by E.J. "Doc" Kreis
Printed by Ambrose Printing Company, Nashville, Tennessee
No part of this publication may be reproduced or transmitted in any form or by any means electronic or mechanical, including photocopying, recording, or any information storage and retrieval system now know or to be invented, without permission in writing from the author, except by a reviewer who wishes to quote brief passages in connection with a written review for inclusion in a magazine, newspaper or broadcast.

Cover and text Design: David G. Lowry
Photo Credit: A. L. James
　　　　　　　Jack Ross
　　　　　　　Bruce Klemens
　　　　　　　Tommy L. Bates
Figure Drawings by C. Hugh Shelton
Additional Graphics by Judy Hall and Suma Clark
Technical Supervisor: Josh Ambrose
Typists: Willma Grant & Galyn Glick
Printed in the United States of America

Edited by
J. P. Montgomery
Director/Honors Program
Professor of English
Middle Tennessee State University
Murfreesboro, Tennessee

ACKNOWLEDGEMENTS

My special thanks to all the many people who have helped make Speed-Strength-Training for Football come to life: to Dr. John Paul Montgomery, my editor and friend; to Josh Ambrose, whose friendship and expert knowledge in preparation is unmatched; to David Lowry, who made the graphics come to life; and to C. Hugh Shelton, who did such a great job on the illustrations; to Wilma Grant, the super typist. Thanks to Judy Hall and Suma Clark for your support, and photographer Jack Ross, who came and helped on a moment's notice.

My special thanks to Strength Coaches Todd Suttles and Matt Riley, who were such a big help to me, and to Coach J. R. Bickerstaff, whose teaching and encouragement never has ended. Thanks, Coach "Boots" Donnelly for the opportunity to return to Strength and Conditioning six years ago and to come to Middle Tennessee State University and see what "could be done with a Strength Coach." To Charles, Ann and Paul McConnell, you are the best.
And a very special thanks to Reebok International Ltd. and Velma Coffey for their tremendous support.

CONTENTS

CHAPTER 1

Introduction 2
Definition of Speed-Strength Training 2
Four Components of Speed-Strength Training 3
    1. Explosive Strength
    2. Starting Strength
    3. Absolute Strength
    4. Reaction Strength
Explosive Strength Component 4
Lower Body Explosiveness 5
Upper Body Explosives 6
Starting Strength Component 6
Absolute Strength Component 7
Reaction Strength Component 9
Coupled Effect of Speed-Strength Training 10

CHAPTER 2-IMPLEMENTING A SPEED-STRENGTH TRAINING PROGRAM

Implementing a Speed-Strength Training Program 12
Year-Round Training Program 12
Nine Steps for Implementing a Program Speed-Strength 13
    Step 1: Period of the Cycle 13
    Step 2: Sequence of Lifting Exercises 14
    Step 3: Number of Repetitions 18
    Step 4: Intensity 23
    Step 5: Frequency of Workouts 23
    Step 6: Warm-Up Routine 24
    Step 7: Relaxation and Flexibility Routine 26
    Step 8: Variability of the Load 27
    Step 9: Number of Exercises 28
Summary 29

CHAPTER 3 - SNATCH AND CLEAN EXERCISES

Snatch and Clean Exercises 32
Lifting Exercises - Full Range Movements 32
The Starting Position and Grips 32
The Grips 32
Snatch Exercises 33
    Exercise 1: Power Snatch 33
    Exercise 2: Split Snatch 35
    Exercise 3: Muscle Snatch 35
    Exercise 4: Olympic Style Snatch (Squat Snatch) 36
    Exercise 5: Snatch Pull 36
    Exercise 6: Hang Snatch 36
    Exercise 7: One-Arm Dumbbell Snatch 38
    Exercise 8: Snatch Pull High Pull 39
Clean Exercises 39
    Exercise 1: Power Clean 40
    Exercise 2: Split Clean 41
    Exercise 3: Muscle Clean 41
    Exercise 4: Olympic Style Clean (Squat Clean) 42
    Exercise 5: Clean Pull 43
    Exercise 6: Hang Clean 43
    Exercise 7: Dumbbell Power Clean 44
    Exercise 8: Clean Pull High Pull 45
Clean and Jerk Exercises 45
    Exercise 1: Clean and Jerk (Two-Part Movement) 46

CHAPTER 4 - PRESS EXERCISES

Press Exercises 50
    Exercise 1: Bench Press 50
    Exercise 2: Incline Bench Press 51
    Exercise 3: Dumbbell Bench Press 52
    Exercise 4: Dumbbell Incline Bench Press 53
    Exercise 5: Behind the Neck Press (Standing) 54
    Exercise 6: Front Press or Military Press (Seated) 54
    Exercise 7: Push Press (or Push Jerk) 55

CHAPTER 5-SQUATS AND LOWER BACK EXERCISES

Squats and Lower Back Exercises 58
    Exercise 1: Back Squat..58
    Exercise 2: Front Squat 59
    Exercise 3: Split Squat..60
    Exercise 4: One-Legged Squat 62
    Exercise 5: Lunge 63
    Exercise 6: Step-Ups/Dumbbells 63
    Exercise 7: Step-Ups/Barbell 64
Hyperextension Exercise 64
Glute Ham Raise Exercise 66
Good Morning Exercises 67
    Exercise 1: Good Morning (Standing) 67
    Exercise 2: Good Morning (Seated/Bent Legs or Straight)..............................68

CHAPTER 6-THE EXTRA EXERCISE ESSENTIALS: GYMNASTIC MOVEMENT AND ABDOMINAL/NECK EXERCISES

Gymnastic Movement Exercises 72
    Exercise 1: Chin-Up...72
    Exercise 2: Parallel Bar Dips 73
    Exercise 3: Ballistic Push-Ups 74
Abdominal and Neck Exercises..74
    Exercise 1: Sit-up with Resistance and Sit-up without Resistance 75
    Exercise 2: Sit-Up Hyperextended 75
    Exercise 3: Hanging Bent Knee/Straight Legs Raise 77
    Exercise 4: Dumbbell Side Bend...78
Neck Exercises 81
    Exercise 1: Wrestler's Bridge 82
    Exercise 2: Neck Harness 82

CHAPTER 7 - PLYOMETRICS - LOWER BODY EXPLOSIVENESS

Lower Body Explosiveness 84
Jumping Drills 85
    Drill 1: Platform Jump 85
    Drill 2: Over the Top Side Jump 86
    Drill 3: Straddle Bench Jump 86
Depth Jump Drills 87
    Drill 4: Depth Jump 88
    Drill 5: Shock Jump 89
    Drill 6: Front Hurdle Hops 90
    Drill 7: Double Leg Hops 91
    Drill 8: Single Leg Hop 91
Squat Jump Drills 92
    Drill 9: Squat Jump 92
Reaction Speed-Strength Plyometric Drills 93
    Drill 1: Hayes Double Leg Top Hops 93
    Drill 2: Hayes Double Leg in the Hole Hops 94
    Drill 3: Hayes Single Leg Top Hops 94
    Drill 4: Hayes Single Leg in the Hole Hops 95
Reaction Speed-Strength Sprinting Drills 95
    Drill 1: Bounds 96
    Drill 2: Running A's 96
    Drill 3: Skips 97

CHAPTER 8 - BALLISTICS - UPPER BODY EXPLOSIVENESS

Medicine Ball Throwing Drills 100
    Drill 1: Standing Overhead Throw and Kneeling 101
    Drill 2: Standing Side Throw 101
    Drill 3: Two-Hand Chest Throw 102
    Drill 4: Sit-Up Throw and Sit-Up Long Throw 103
    Drill 5: Underhand/Back Overhead Throw 104
    Drill 6: Bench Press Throw 104
    Drill 7: Press Throw 105
Ballistic Push-Up 105
    Drill 8: Ballistic Push-Up 106
Weight Throws 107

CHAPTER 9-EVALUATION AND TESTING OF SPEED-STRENGTH TRAINING

Evaluation and Testing of Speed-Strength Training..110
Suggestions on When to Evaluate the Test 110
Running Races...111
    Races 1, 2, 3: 40-60- & 100 yard Dashes 112
    Race 4: 880-yard Run 112
Reaction - Speed Drills...113
    Drill 1: Line Touch...113
    Drill 2: Figure Eight..114
    Drill 3: Four Corner...115
Strength 116
Jumping...117
    Drill 1: Vertical Jump..118
    Drill 2: Standing Long Jump...118
    Drill 3: Standing Triple Jump..119
Medicine Ball Throws 119
    Drill 1: Seated long Throw 120
    Drill 2: Standing Long Throw 121
    Drill 3: Standing Back Overhead Long Throw..121
Body Measurements..122
Self-Evaluation Training Journal..122

CHAPTER 10-MOTIVATIONAL TECHNIQUES IN SPEED-STRENGTH TRAINING

Motivational Techniques in Speed-Strength Training..130
Use of Goals..130
Trainer and Coach as Motivator 131
Promoting Speed-Strength Training 131
Photographs 131
Record Boards 131
Monthly Progress Reports...132
Testing..
132
Team Contest..132
Mottos and Quotas...132
Special Awards..132

GLOSSARY
....134

REFERENCES
....143

Finally, to my wife Danielle,
my daughter Taylor
and my son E. J.,
who are my Speed-Strength,
you made it all worth the journey.

In Speed-Strength,

E. J. "Doc" Kreis

In memory of
David Gilberto Lora
whose spirit is still with us
in his pictures throughout
Speed-Strength Training for Football.

FORWARD

In all the world of sports, SPEED is king. In any sport the athlete who is able to consistently perform each and every movement with instantaneous maximum force output will dominate his peers. There is only one way of acquiring this ability -- through application of integrative science. Doc Kreis' book on *SPEED-STRENGTH TRAINING FOR FOOTBALL* is a unique and masterful example on integrative thinking.

Dr. Fred Hatfield ("Dr. Squat")--
World Powerlifting Champion, World Record Holder and Author

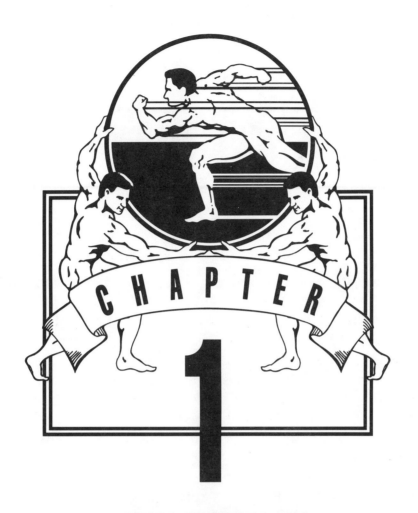

INTRODUCTION

"How do you want to be remembered?"
Football Coach Ed Bunio

INTRODUCTION

The idea of what is needed to produce maximum performance training routines for football players revolves around what would be most productive for optimal gains. In the 1960's Soviet Union coaches and scientists coined a new phrase for power. They called power "speed-strength." The introduction of the concept of speed-strength training has allowed athletes to progress in the Eastern Block countries and to surpass athletic development in the West. Because of the level of competition and the conditioning of football players today, athletes, trainers and coaches are searching for progressive and aggressive weight-training methods and techniques. Success in football calls for the combined efforts of speed to strength. What has happened in the development of football players has been at the extreme—either too much strength and not enough speed training or the effect of speed without any method of obtaining strength. The end effort is that the athlete is only one-half better than when he started.

The fusion of a speed and strength training program can produce the greatest amount of power and speed possible. This combination of speed-strength training with the regular conditioning programs has the potential to revolutionize the play of any football player. Speed-strength training for football is a designed year-round, planned program model for the athlete. Implementing an unplanned program, with no blueprint or understanding of what foundation base is needed, is only inviting failure. To invite success, Dr. Verhoshansky, a Soviet trainer, advises the coach to consider that achievement is dependent on the relationship of speed's co-existence with the development of strength. The incorporation of a speed-strength training program is the cornerstone for championship football.

DEFINITION OF SPEED-STRENGTH TRAINING

Speed-strength training is defined as the combination of maximum speed incorporated in maximum strength, thus producing the greatest amount of power. A speed-strength training program should first be constructed in accordance with the principle of a gradually increasing work intensity and, second, be combined with technique training to develop the athlete for the capacity to execute his position at full exertion. Performance improvement of players at the professional football level, representing the highest state of speed-strength mastery, is determined primarily by increasing each individual's special-specific work capacity. This is also an essential operating condition for improving the athlete's ability in the competitive situation, game or practice.

FOUR COMPONENTS OF SPEED-STRENGTH TRAINING

The combining of speed and strength into a training program can be divided into four components. The four components of speed-strength are:
1. Explosive strength-the greatest amount of force developed in a time frame;
2. Starting strength-the measurement of how fast and forceful the athletic motion is at the beginning;
3. Absolute strength-the maximum one can lift, regardless of the time chosen to perform it in;
4. Reaction strength-the speed in which the initial body movement causes an opposite and increased reaction from the second movement that occurs to the follow-through.

Dr. Verhoshansky lists the first three components as the foundation of speed-strength training and essential for peak athletic performance. The fourth is what the author believes to be the final component that incorporates the total development of the speed-strength training model for football.

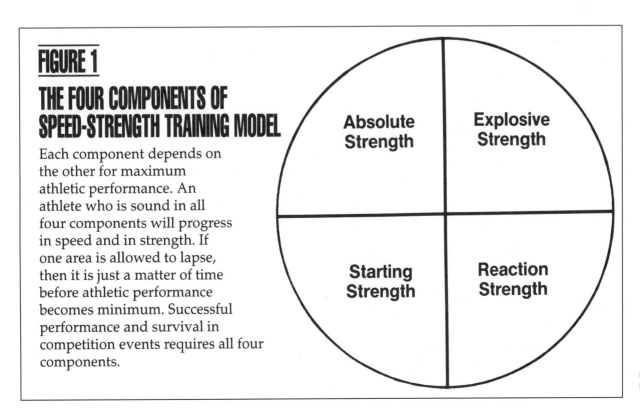

FIGURE 1
THE FOUR COMPONENTS OF SPEED-STRENGTH TRAINING MODEL

Each component depends on the other for maximum athletic performance. An athlete who is sound in all four components will progress in speed and in strength. If one area is allowed to lapse, then it is just a matter of time before athletic performance becomes minimum. Successful performance and survival in competition events requires all four components.

EXPLOSIVE STRENGTH COMPONENT

Of the four principles of speed-strength training, the most important is explosive strength. Explosive strength is the maximum amount of power developed in a certain time frame (Figure 2). A key to explosive strength is to explode in the beginning or where the force is maximum for acceleration to finish or repeat an exercise or athletic movement. Explosive strength is developed by using weight-lifting exercises (Figure 3), jumping (Figure 4 and 4A) and throwing exercise (Figure 5) drills of an explosive nature, which are now known in the sports world as plyometrics and ballistics.

The secret of explosive strength lies in transferring the specific movement to the athletic skill. If blocking a defensive man by an offensive player requires the explosive movement of moving from stance to contact to follow-through, then the understanding of the upper body and lower body speed-strength training requires specially designed exercises, drill method and technique.

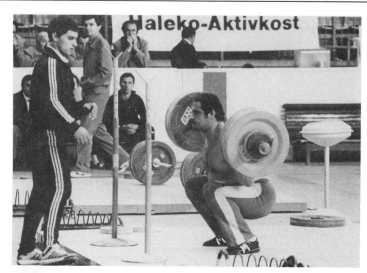

FIGURE 2
Explosive Strength-the Explosiveness that will occur from the upward movement in the Back Squat

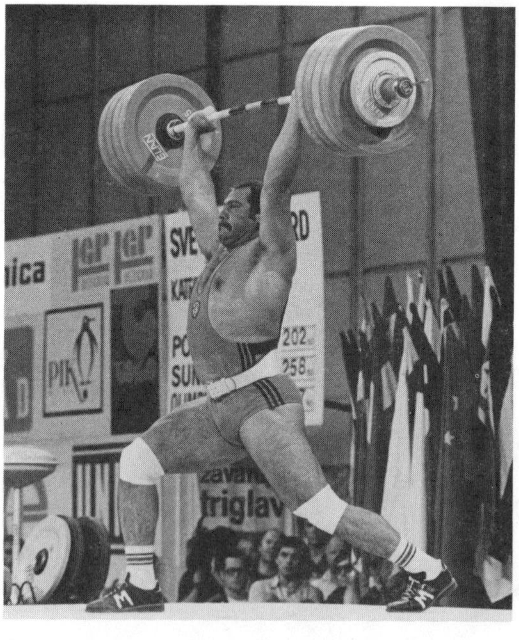

FIGURE 3
Weight Lifting using Explosive Strength to complete the Clean and Jerk

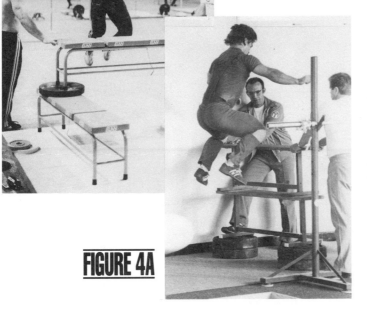

FIGURE 4

Pylometric Jumping using Explosive Strength

FIGURE 4A

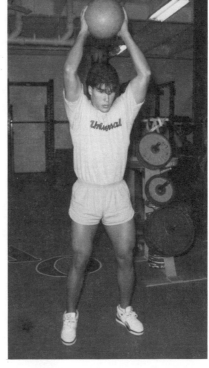

FIGURE 5

Ballistic Throwing using Explosive Strength

LOWER BODY EXPLOSIVENESS

Today, speed is even more high-priced than ever before. We are no longer faced with the good, little fast guy, but the good, fast, big guy who does it all.

The key to football training is the lower body-explosive strength in dealing with plyometrics explosion of the legs, hips, back and glutes. The lower body is refined and strengthened by jump exercises. These jumps are described as jumping on top of, jumping over, jumping around, jumping up and jumping out. The depth jumps, whether with one leg, both legs, single or double, are described as jumping off, step-offs and altitude jumps. The depth jumps are the best and most effective method for developing this quick, explosive strength along with the proper speed-strength training program to accompany it. The hops and bounds bring to the athlete the skill transferable factors of balance, coordination and dexterity of plyometrics.

UPPER BODY EXPLOSIVES

The more popular lift today in football weight training seems to be the bench press. Too many football players who train this particular lift seem to do very little to assist the development of speed. In speed-strength the upper body ballistics and the principles of explosive strength are enhanced. Too many football players become one-dimensional. What happens in their training is that they have no other option than just loading the bar and letting it go. Upper body explosiveness can achieve the attainment of absolute strength and add speed to improve the explosiveness of movement. For the football player the importance of upper body explosive strength is vital in the required football activities of the arms, shoulders, chest and back.

STARTING STRENGTH COMPONENT

Starting strength is the second component of speed-strength training. Starting strength and explosive strength work together very closely, yet their values are different. Starting strength is a measure of how fast and forceful the movement is at the beginning (Figure 6). What quickly comes to mind as an example of starting strength is the tremendous sprinting start of Ben Johnson of Canada in the finals in Rome, Italy, in 1987. His start was one of the greatest ever witnessed in track and field history, and his time proved this fact. With little more than body resistance, the running or sprinting start is a foundation base for starting strength. Dr. Fred Hatfield and Dr. Michael Yessis state in their excellent book <u>Plyometric Training</u> that the lighter the implement the athlete moves and the shorter the distance, the more starting strength he acquires; the heavier the resistance and the longer the distance, the more important his explosive strength becomes.

Starting is the individual's instantaneous ability to recruit as many muscle cells as possible. The first key of starting strength is the ability to concentrate and gather for the initial effort. An example that exemplifies starting strength in the lifts is the starting position of the Olympic snatch lift. The individual athlete should be able to gather for the intended movement and then allow the second chain reaction of explosion to reaction strength to occur. Starting strength is the ability to get maximum muscle explosion instantly. It should be built on a foundation of great absolute strength. The take-off and the quick-strength are both names of the component—starting strength. Starting strength is a measure of how fast and forceful the movement is at the beginning. An example is an offensive lineman firing off the line of scrimmage and making contact with the defense player. This is a picture of starting and explosive strength made visible by working together and following through with the starting and explosive speed-strength. Starting strength and acceleration are dependent upon each other. One of the best ways to develop the starting strength component is by coaching the athlete to make the maximal effort at the beginning of any speed-strength training exercise or drill.

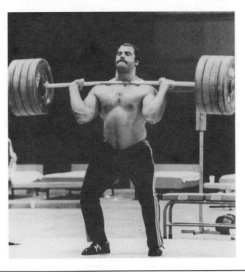

FIGURE 6
Starting strength to an Overhead Press

ABSOLUTE STRENGTH COMPONENT

The third component of speed-strength is absolute strength. Ever since Milo, a Greek athlete of much fame and Olympic magnitude, lifted his first baby calf, man has been infatuated with how much he can lift. Milo would carry this newborn calf upon his shoulders daily. At first, there was the task of lifting and positioning the animal; then Milo had to walk the prescribed distance for this training regime. As the calf grew, the weight also increased, but as the story goes, so did Milo's strength grow along with the size of the growing calf.

Milo's search for strength led in the direction of absolute strength training. This principle is based on how much one can lift in a single repetition or attempt to lift in a given exercise. It is a measure of maximum strength. For the beginning weight trainer, how much weight lifted in a single try is not the factor of importance, but what is important is the proper technique and method.

For the beginner, the attitude is too often one of trying to lift too much too soon. Without proper coaching of technique and method to guarantee that the exercise is performed correctly, the factors of absolute strength only stand to hinder the football player's training. The beginner needs to lay a solid foundation for the development of speed-strength training. The program should entail major assistance of gymnastic movements — dips, chin-ups, pull-ups, push-ups—to specific running and reaction development drills — knee lifts, bounds, and stride and frequency drills (See Figure 7).

For the intermediate athlete, absolute strength starts to become a factor in the training program. The intermediate athlete should build into his program a check and balance so that he can periodically see what progress has been made. Many young athletes associate strength and speed gains as the only factors of pounds lifted. This leads the intermediate athlete to try too much or try to keep up with someone who is further along in his training. Standards are important, but only from the standpoint of records of individual accomplishment. What is most important is that the athlete be supervised by a successful and well-instructed coach or trainer who can advise him of what can be accomplished with intelligent hard work and time. Too much programming for absolute strength is the same as too many timed races for running and sprinting. The athlete never gets to learn how to develop his strength or speed because he never is allowed to train. An important factor to consider with the intermediate lifter is practicing a specific movement that encompasses the transfer from one area of sport to another; this emphasis demands more sets and repetition with more training time.

Absolute strength training for the advanced athlete is at a period of time where scheduled practice and development of speed-strength movements are totally involved with the training program. Now is the importance of when absolute strength is to be reached and peak athletic performance is developed—the understanding of when to attempt 90 percent, 95 percent and 100 percent, a totally new personal record (PR). This is absolute strength. *Absolute is the total effort, not just the attempted but the accomplished. That is what one strives to project in peak performance.*

The most common questions from advanced athletes regarding absolute strength are: When should these peaks be tried and how often? What effect will the attempt of absolute strength have on the body and what will the period of recovery and restoration be? Answers to these questions will vary from individual to individual—understanding how bodies best function and what factors of limitations one must face. Again, as with the beginner and the intermediate athlete, too much too often will not only lead to possible enthusiasm failure, but will also injure muscles and dampen the spirit.

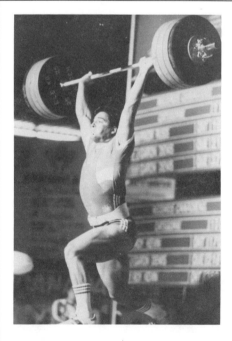

FIGURE 7

Absolute Strength exemplified in the Clean and Jerk

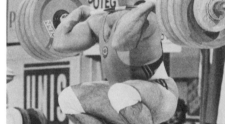

FIGURE 8

The Effort of Absolute Strength

To many well-trained athletes, absolute strength has different meanings; one is that every repetition, regardless of when or where it is performed on the schedule, is treated as the absolute repetition or attempt. This kind of positive thinking and attitude encourages positive motivation and positive habits that trainers and coaches hope will endure through the football season (See Figure 8).

REACTION STRENGTH COMPONENT

The fourth component of speed-strength is reaction strength. Reaction strength is defined as the speed in which the initial body movement causes an opposite and increased reaction from the second movement that occurs to the follow-through. An example is when a football player is charging off the line of scrimmage, adjusting his body position to gain advantage of placing his body under the oncoming defender. The player's reaction strength increases from the second movement to the follow-through that is required in most skills needed in playing football (Figure 9).

Many athletes use reaction strength in defining quickness. Friction and acceleration are key elements of reaction strength. The development of force in pushing off or pulling aids in the total attitude of reaction. A few years ago, in working with Assistant Basketball Coach John Bostick at Vanderbilt University, I observed that he used a drill that he named action-reaction. The drill consisted of one player moving and the other player facing the individual reacting to his movement. The drill only lasted a few seconds, but the amount of force and concentration exerted by the players points to the base of reaction strength—*that the components of speed-strength occurring in an athlete's training exemplify the importance of "the greater the strength, the greater the speed" of the athlete.* The reaction strength component (meaning two movements in one) can best be developed by use of combination lifts. By changing movement to movements, the muscles are given greater direction for growth and speed-strength development.

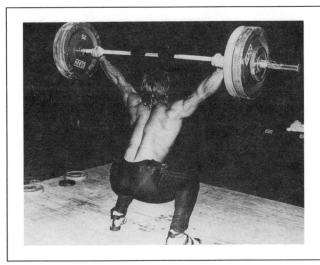

FIGURE 9

Reaction Strength - Allows the player's Reaction Strength to increase from Second Movement to the Follow-Through

COUPLED EFFECT OF SPEED-STRENGTH TRAINING

The four components of speed-strength training, -- absolute, explosive, starting, and reaction strength -- are only as good as the "coupled effect" of the combined skills needed for the overall development of the football player. The skills of blocking, tackling, catching and running are required as methods and techniques to be improved as the player's skill level improves.

Dr. Michael Yessis gives an example using the football lineman who has the ability to bench press five hundred pounds. He says that, ". . . doesn't mean he will be able to stop a charging opponent in a particular manner. In other words, having the strength needed must be 'coupled' with the skill (motor task) to be executed." By identifying specific skills needed in football, the athletic coach or trainer can better determine numbers of repetitions, sets and kinds of series for specific exercises planned.

The use of speed-strength training helps maintain the delicate balance of the four components of speed strength. Author John P. Jesse states that "because strength is easier to develop than other qualities, athletes spend more time in developing great strength than in developing the speed, timing and balance that would put their strength to greater use in performance." *Speed-strength training for football is about building the best football body*. By understanding the difference between body building, power lifting and weight lifting, you understand the process of developing a faster and stronger athlete. Still football comes down to blocking, tackling, running, kicking, catching and throwing. If you execute these skills more effectively, you improve and so does your team. This leaves us with the final introductory statement that "with speed-strength training, the best athletic performances are yet to come."

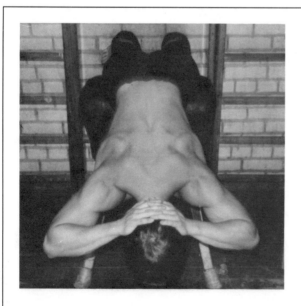
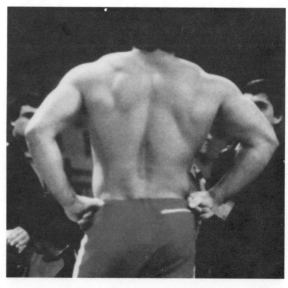

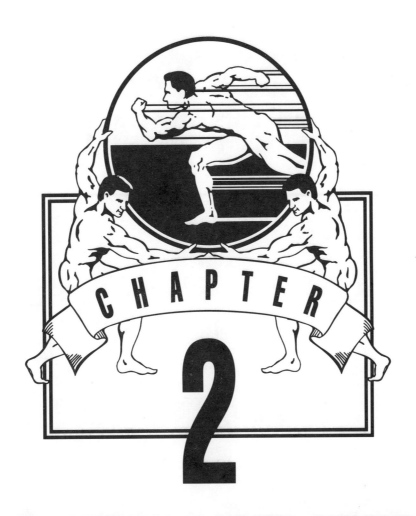

CHAPTER 2

IMPLEMENTING A SPEED-STRENGTH TRAINING PROGRAM

"If I do not practice one day, I know it. If I do not practice the next, the orchestra knows it. If I do not practice the third day, the whole world knows it."
Ignace Paderewski
Polish Pianist

IMPLEMENTING A SPEED-STRENGTH TRAINING PROGRAM

To achieve the necessary response to training, the implementation of a speed-strength program with many variables is necessary. These variables will include: volume, number, sequences of exercises, number of repetitions per set, frequency of workouts, variability of the load, number of exercises and tempo at which the performed exercises are carried out in training. *This chapter defines the placement of these variables within the year-round training program so the athlete can give form and meaning to a master plan that ensures success.*

YEAR-ROUND TRAINING PROGRAM

The periodization phases–preparatory, competitive, and transition–allow for well-planned and well-executed programs. The next step is implementing these phases with the four components of speed-strength training - absolute, explosive, starting, and reaction. By incorporating the three phases of periodization, the athlete, coach or trainer can make decisions to handle the development of the annual training cycle of speed and strength training (See Table 2).

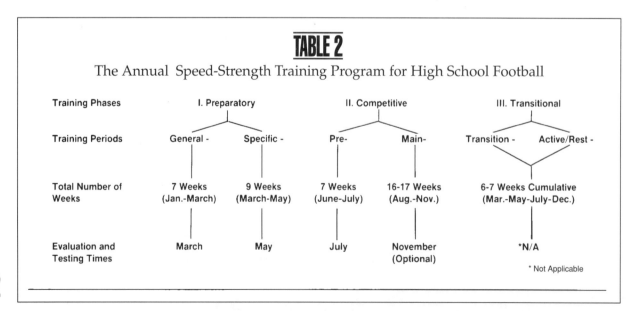

TABLE 2
The Annual Speed-Strength Training Program for High School Football

Training Phases	I. Preparatory		II. Competitive		III. Transitional	
Training Periods	General -	Specific -	Pre-	Main-	Transition -	Active/Rest -
Total Number of Weeks	7 Weeks (Jan.-March)	9 Weeks (March-May)	7 Weeks (June-July)	16-17 Weeks (Aug.-Nov.)	6-7 Weeks Cumulative (Mar.-May-July-Dec.)	
Evaluation and Testing Times	March	May	July	November (Optional)	*N/A	

* Not Applicable

NINE STEPS FOR IMPLEMENTING A PROGRAM

In implementing a speed-strength training program, the essential elements are the lifting exercises, the plyometric and ballistics. The nine steps in which a speed-strength training program is implemented are as follows: (1) period of the cycle, (2) sequence of the lifting exercises, (3) number of repetitions, (4) intensity, (5) frequency of workouts, (6) warm-up routine, (7) relaxation and flexibility routine, (8) variability of the load and (9) number of exercises.

By utilizing the nine steps, the athlete, trainer or coach will have incorporated the four components of speed-strength–explosive, starting, absolute, and reaction, thus providing the key elements and foundation for a successful, winning edge.

STEP 1: PERIOD OF THE CYCLE

Incorporating the three phases of periodization into the annual planning cycle of the speed-strength training program involves blocking off the amount of time necessary for the development of the football player during each phase. By listing the three phases, the coach becomes aware of the amount of time (number of workouts) and the amount of repetitions needed to carry out the speed-strength program. Football coaches use similar systems in scheduling daily football practices during the course of the season and in preparation for the season. This planning of the annual cycle should be no different.

In the *preparatory phase*, the preparatory cycle is subdivided into two periods, *general* and *specific*, and includes the amount of time one will spend during the preparatory phase during the spring of the school year and during the early summer out-of-school months. During the preparatory phase while the athletes are in school, the training time (total minutes) is considered because of the amount of time after school that is available, along with the total number of training days available.

The *competitive phase* is divided into two periods, *pre-competitive* and *main competitive*. The main-competitive period is the time of early summer before the start of the season and fall of the school year. The amount of strength training is placed in priority of a two-a-day or three-a-day football practice in preparation for the football season to begin. As the number of main-competitive practices remaining becomes less, the practice time before the first game or the opening game coincides with the return to the classrooms and the opening of the school year. The focus now shifts to game-week preparation and the main-competitive period.

In the main-competitive period, the weekly game preparation is now a routine in itself. For example:
1. Friday–game day
2. Saturday–injury and condition report (possible speed-strength day)
3. Sunday–coaches' review and grading of the game film from Friday night
4. Monday–scouting report and practice (possible speed-strength training day)
5. Tuesday–heavy practice and game plan script (possible speed-strength training day)
6. Wednesday–emphasis on game preparation (possible speed-strength training day)
7. Thursday–final preparation and detailed game run through.

Friday marks the day or night of the game, bringing to a close the weekly game preparation during the main-competitive period. It is very important to place the seven steps into the main-competitive period so as to create the best situation.

The *transitional phase* is subdivided into the *transition* and *active rest period*. The first part of the transitional phase is the transition period. The transition periods occur at the end of the fall football season, at the conclusion for the general preparatory period, and at the end of spring training or the specific preparatory period. These three breaks in the transitional phase action allow for time away from coaches, school, teammates and a chance to get a change of scenery away from the training and the sport. This helps in restoring enthusiasm, spirit and attitude and allows for one to reflect on what was accomplished. This is important for football players and equally important for football coaches. The amount of stress–physically, mentally and emotionally–can be the most detrimental factor to a coach's well-being. The second phase of transition is the period of active rest. Too many programs refer to time off simply as the time in which athletes spend weeks and months out of training. The maximum amount of transition period away should be no more than fourteen days and no less than three. The use of active rest should not be a full week schedule, but should allow the football player a progressive number of days back in speed-strength training and a progressive number of days with sports activities of a different nature, such as basketball, swimming, soccer, handball, tennis or racquetball. Then the athlete should progress to the speed-strength training of light or medium lifting and light reaction-speed until the implemented time of training is begun.

STEP 2: SEQUENCE OF LIFTING EXERCISES

Vorobyev, in an excerpt from his book *Weightlifting,* outlines the order of exercises in each training phase as the fastest movement first.

The following are twelve speed-strength categories of lifting exercises and the sequence.

First Exercises: Snatch
1. Power snatch
2. Split snatch
3. Muscle snatch
4. Snatch–Olympic style
5. Snatch pull (can also be heavy movement, determined by intensity of the load)
6. Dumbbell snatch
7. One arm dumbell snatch
8. Snatch pull - High pull

Second Exercises: Clean
1. Power clean
2. Split clean
3. Muscle clean
4. Clean–Olympic style
5. Clean pull (can be determined by intensity of load)
6. Hang clean–not a complete movement
7. Dumbbell Power clean
8. Clean pull - high pull

Third Exercises: Press
1. Bench press
2. Incline bench press
3. Dumbbell bench press

4. Dumbbell incline bench press
5. Behind neck press
6. Front press or military press
7. Push press
8. Narrow grip bench press

Fourth Exercises: Squat
1. Back squat
2. Front squat
3. Split squat
4. One-legged squat
5. Lunge
6. Step-ups/Dumbbells
7. Step-ups/Barbells

Fifth Exercises: Good Morning
1. Squat style
2. Straight-legged
3. Seated (straight-legged and bent leg)

Sixth Exercise: Combination Lifts
1. Clean and Jerk
2. Snatch and Squat
3. Squat and Jerk

Seventh Exercises: Jerk
1. From the rack
2. From the clean
3. Push jerk

Eighth Exercises: Hyperextension
1. Hyperextension
2. Russian twist/stick
3. Russian twist/medicine ball

Ninth Exercise: Glute Ham Raise
1. Glute ham raise
2. Glute ham raise sit-ups
3. Glute ham alternate dumbbell twist

Tenth Exercises: Gymnastics
1. Chin-up
2. Dip
3. Ballistics push-up

Eleventh Exercises: Abdominal
1. Sit-up–weighted straight legs
2. Hyper sit-up–weighted
3. Chin-up leg raise

Twelfth Exercises: Neck
1. Wrestler's bridge
2. Pulling-movements
3. Neck harness

The athlete, trainer or coach can choose from twelve different categories of lifting exercises, as well as select from plyometrics and ballistics training drills. How to fit these exercises into different sequence and/or order is discussed in Step 9.

Sequencing of the preparatory phase (See Table 3) Each exercise is listed in the order of speed to strength, incorporating the four components of speed-strength training for the preparatory phase. Thus, by using the same exercise worked in a different motion, the duplication of snatching, cleaning, pressing and squatting every day is possible.

Sequencing of the competitive phase (see Tables 4 and 5) Because of the intensity of the two-a-day practice, the speed-strength training program should be kept to a minimum number of key movements. The maximum number of exercises and the sequence should not be over three. This takes into consideration the factors of recovery and restoration for the athlete necessary during these practice days.

TABLE 3
Exercises of Speed-Strength Training

Snatches	Cleans	Squats	Presses
1. Power snatch	1. Power clean	1. Back squat	1. Bench press
2. Split snatch	2. Split clean	2. Front squat	2. Incline bench press
3. Muscle snatch	3. Muscle clean	3. Split squat	3. Dumbbell bench press
4. Olympic-style snatch	4. Olympic-style clean	4. One-legged squat	4. Dumbbell incline bench press
5. Snatch pull	5. Clean pull	5. Lunge	5. Behind neck press
6. Hang snatch	6. Hang clean	6. Step-ups/dumbbells	6. Front press or military press
7. One-arm dumbbell snatch	7. Dumbbell power clean	7. Step-ups/barbell	7. Push press or push jerk
8. Snatch pull-high pull	8. Clean pull-high pull		

Good Mornings	Combination Lifts		Jerks
1. Squat style	1. Clean and jerk		1. Clean and jerk
2. Seated	Classical olympic style		2. Jerk from stand
a. Straight legs	2. Front squat plus push press		3. Push-jerk
b. Bent legs	3. Back squat plus behind		
	neck press		
	4. Front squat plus jerk		
	5. Snatch plus squat		

Hyperextensions	Glute Ham Raises	Gymnastics Movements	Neck
1. Hyperextension	1. Glute ham raises	1. Chin-up	1. Wrestlers-bridge
2. Russian twist/stick	2. Glute ham raise sit-ups	2. Dip	2. Pulling-movement
3. Russian twist/medicine ball	3. Glute ham alternative dumbbell twist	3. Ballistic push-up	3. Head harness

Abdominal	Plyometrics	Ballistics	
1. Sit-up with weight	1. Jumps	1. Medicine ball throws	
2. Hyperextension sit-up	2. Depth jumps	2. Push-up	
3. Crunch	3. Hops	3. Weight throws	
4. Chin-up leg raise	4. Reaction speed-strength		
5. Sit-up	5. Reaction speed-strength sprinting		
6. Seated, behind neck weight twist			
7. Medicine ball sit-up			

The main-competitive period is the football season. The idea is not just to maintain a level of speed-strength, but to build more foundation into the structure of speed-strength development. The increase in absolute strength will be minimal due to the energy output of game play, but an increase in explosive, starting and reaction strength should be achievable. The coaches can decide what they want to do, practice before implementing any speed-strength training or speed-strength training before practice. Football coaches can opt to use certain speed-strength warm-up drills as the players report to practice. Examples are: (1) one-legged squats as an excellent thigh and knee warm-up, (2) glute ham raises as an excellent hamstring warm-up exercise, (3) dips and/or chin-ups, (4) sit-ups and (5) ballistic throws. *Speed-strength training scheduled with practice is the key to having a winning edge and an aggressive program.* In Table 5, Saturday is the first day of the new week; and if any lifting is done on Saturday or Sunday, the warm-up routine is placed in effect. Then on the following day, they are off.

This helps football teams in the recovery and restoration of the players.

TABLE 4
Main Competitive Days and Sequence of Exercises

DAY 1 SATURDAY	DAY 2 SUNDAY	DAY 3 MONDAY	DAY 4 TUESDAY	DAY 5 WEDNESDAY	DAY 6 THURSDAY	DAY 7 FRIDAY
WARM-UP ROUTINE	OFF	POWER CLEAN	MUSCLE SNATCH	POWER SNATCH	DETAIL	GAME DAY
POWER SNATCH	OFF	SNATCH PULL	CLEAN AND JERK	POWER CLEAN	OFF	
CLEAN PULL	OFF	FRONT SQUAT	SPLIT SQUAT	ONE-LEGGED SQUAT	GAME PREPARATION	
BACK SQUAT	OFF	NARROW GRIP BENCH PRESS	DUMBBELL INCLINE	BENCH PRESS		
BENCH PRESS	OFF	GYMNASTICS MOVEMENT	BENCH PRESS	HYPEREXTENSION		
GYMNASTICS MOVEMENT	OFF	PLYOMETRICS	GOOD MORNING	PLYOMETRICS		
BALLISTICS	OFF	NECK	GYMNASTICS MOVEMENT	BALLISTICS		
ABDOMINAL	OFF	ABDOMINAL	NECK	NECK		
RELAXATION/FLEXIBILITY	OFF	RELAXATION/FLEXIBILITY	ABDOMINAL	ABDOMINAL		
			RELAXATION/FLEXIBILITY	RELAXATION/FLEXIBILITY		

TABLE 5
Preparatory Phase- Multi Days and Sequence of Exercise

DAY 1 MONDAY	DAY 2 TUESDAY	DAY 3 WEDNESDAY	DAY 4 THURSDAY	DAY 5 FRIDAY
WARM-UP ROUTINE	WARM-UP ROUTINE	WARM-UP ROUTINE	WARM-UP ROUTINE	WARM-UP ROUTINE
POWER SNATCH	SPLIT SNATCH	MUSCLE SNATCH	POWER SNATCH	SPLIT SNATCH
SPLIT CLEAN	POWER CLEAN	CLEAN PULL	CLEAN AND JERK	POWER CLEAN
PUSH PRESS	BEHIND NECK PRESS/SEATED	JERK FROM STAND	BEHIND NECK PRESS	PUSH PRESS
BACK SQUAT	FRONT SQUAT	SPLIT SQUAT	BACK SQUAT	FRONT SQUAT
BENCH PRESS	NARROW GRIP BENCH PRESS	INCLINE D.B. BENCH PRESS	BENCH PRESS	NARROW GRIP BENCH PRESS
HYPEREXTENSION	GOOD MORNING	HYPEREXTENSION	GOOD MORNING	HYPEREXTENSION
PLYOMETRICS	PLYOMETRICS	PLYOMETRICS	PLYOMETRICS	GYMNASTICS MOVEMENT
GYMNASTICS MOVEMENT	GYMNASTICS MOVEMENT	GYMNASTICS MOVEMENT	GYMNASTICS MOVEMENT	PLYOMETRICS
BALLISTICS	BALLISTICS	BALLISTICS	BALLISTICS	BALLISTICS
NECK	NECK	NECK	NECK	NECK
ABDOMINAL	ABDOMINAL	ABDOMINAL	ABDOMINAL	ABDOMINAL
RELAXATION/FLEXIBILITY	RELAXATION/FLEXIBILITY	RELAXATION/FLEXIBILITY	RELAXATION/FLEXIBILITY	RELAXATION/FLEXIBILITY

Sequencing of the transitional phase. The transition period and the active rest period are promoted to allow the athletes to regroup physically, mentally and emotionally. The following activities are suggested as examples of the active rest period:

Monday
Run 440-yards--medium speed
Stretch and loosen up
One-legged squat
Standing long jump
Snatch pull
Back Squat
Behind neck press
Gymnastic movement--chin-up
Sit-up
Long, slow distance--12 minutes

Tuesday
Play basketball or racquetball or swim for 45 minutes to 1 hour

Wednesday
Long, slow distance--12 minutes

Thursday
Run 440-yards--medium speed
Stretch and loosen up One-legged squat
Box jump (jump on box)
Power clean
Bench press
Front squat
Gymnastic movement--dip
Sit-up
Long, slow distance--12 minutes

Friday
A sport activity for 1 hour

STEP 3: NUMBER OF REPETITIONS

The number of repetitions (volume) depends upon the percentage of weight that is being used per training workout, thus getting the standards and guidelines which set up the maximum count of repetitions that can be done in each exercise.

The classifications of the athletes will give volume boundaries (number of repetitions) geared to the level of each player's ability:

Pre Phase and Pre-Competitive Period					Main Competitive Period
Beginning	=	Number of Reps	18		12
Intermediate	=	Number of Reps	24		18
Advanced	=	Number of Reps	30		24
Elite	=	Number of Reps	36		28

By limiting the number of repetitions (volume), the athlete gains speed-strength throughout the year.

In preparing the volume and the intensity (amount of weight) of the exercise that is to be trained, the key to developing greater athletic success is to get the most out of each training session. By incorporating the "Training Load Cycle" (see following pages) and the labeling systems of S=Small, M=Medium and B=Big, the planner will progress with the desired training zone load. Regardless of the number of work-outs per week, the "change" to the training-goal allows the exercise to not have a plateauing or leveling off effect. By using the labeling system, the zones become easy to arrange so that maximum results will be made and each work-out receives a value.

In the nine-week and seven-week training zone load cycle, the chart illustrates the two work-outs per week. This then gives the athlete more room to develop over the two different weekly cycles. Work-out days, Monday and Thursday, in a week are in the nine-week cycle; you can see Monday as S=Small and Thursday as M=Medium.

The idea is to "not put any three zones back to back," thus allowing for speed-strength restoration to occur. By using and structuring the S-M-B training zone load cycle, the creative athlete, coach and trainer can put many interesting and different combinations together and provide maximum gains in speed-strength training (See Example A).

SPEED-STRENGTH COACHING TIPS

(1) If two training zones are the same, the next work-out zone will vary.

> **EXAMPLE**
> S-M
> M-B
> MM
> B-S
> Change in different zone

(2) This variation allows the plan to be creative for the individual as well as team training routine during the different training periods.
(3) The designer should watch and protect against "overtraining" and "undertraining."
(4) Adjustments and flexibility can make change and redirection occur for maximum speed-strength gains.

In the preparatory phase and pre-competitive period, the maximum number of repetitions per exercise is 18-36, and in the main-competitive period, the total number of repetitions per exercise is 12-28. Having limits on the amount of repetitions allowed during a training time safeguards against over-training and/or undertraining (Table 6B, see page 22). The following are examples of the preparatory phase or pre-competitive period (limit of repetitions is twenty-four, and bottom number represents repetitions):

EXAMPLE

Power snatch $\frac{50}{6}$ $\frac{55}{5}$ $\frac{60}{5}$ 2   Repetitions: 21

6 + 5 + 10 = 21

Split clean $\frac{55}{5}$ $\frac{65}{4}$ $\frac{70}{3}$ 4   Repetitions: 21

5 + 4 + 12 = 21

Push press $\frac{50}{5}$ $\frac{55}{5}$ $\frac{65}{4}$ 3   Repetitions: 22

5 + 5 + 12 = 22

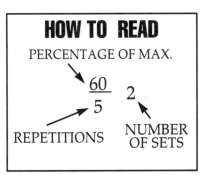

EXAMPLE A

ONE WEEK/FOUR-DAY TRAINING PLAN WITH LOADING ZONES
NON-COMPETITIVE PERIOD

WEEK #1

EXERCISES	MONDAY	TUESDAY	WEDNESDAY	THURSDAY	FRIDAY
Warm-up Routine	Train	Train		Train	Train
Clean Pull	B			B	
Snatch Pull		M			S
Snatch	M			M	
Split Snatch	S	S		M	M
Power Clean	S			M	M
Clean and Jerk		B		M	M
Jerk from Rack	S			M	
Back Squat	S			S	B
Front Squat		M	"Team Sports" Activity Workout	S	B
Bench Press	M			M	B
Closed-Grip Bench Press		S			B
Dips		Train			Train
Chin-Ups	Train			Train	
Plyometrics	Reaction Speed-Strength (Hayes Hops)	Speed-Strength Running Drills		Reaction Speed-Strength (Hayes Hops)	Speed-Strength Running Drills
Ballistics (Medicine Ball)	Standing Drills	Floor Drills		Standing Drills	Floor Drills
Weighted Sit-Ups	Train	Train		Train	Train
Relaxation and Flexibility Routine	Train	Train		Train	Train

NOTE: Special thanks to Jerry Tubbs for his input.

This review should help in implementing the exercises the coach would like to use, and by referring to the three examples, you can see that each was within the limit. Next is an example of the main-competition period (limit of repetitions is eighteen):

EXAMPLE

Power snatch	$\frac{50}{5}$	$\frac{55}{6}$ 2		Repetitions: 17
Clean pull	$\frac{55}{6}$ 3			Repetitions: 18
Back squat	$\frac{60}{6}$	$\frac{65}{5}$	$\frac{70}{4}$	Repetitions: 15

All three examples have stayed within the eighteen-repetition limits per exercise of the main-competitive period.

Nine-Week Training Zone Load Cycle

Number of Weeks	Workouts Per Week	
	First	Second
1	S	M
2	M	M
3	B	S
4	M	B
5	S	M
6	B	M
7	M	S
8	S	M
9	Evaluation and Testing	

Seven-Week Training Zone Load Cycle

Number of Weeks	Workouts Per Week	
	First	Second
1	M	M
2	S	M
3	S	B
4	S	M
5	B	S
6	M	M
7	Evaluation and Testing	

S - Small; M - Medium; B - Big

In planning a routine of speed-strength training, a natural time factor should be built in so that each exercise has a limited number of total repetitions, as well as a maximum number per exercise. *The sequence of exercises includes no warm-up sets; each exercise moves the athlete in a progressive direction that prepares him for the next exercise.* The listed percentages, sets and repetitions are the work-out program and have no additional or extra lifting. Another factor is the limit of repetitions per set. Again, the training zone (Table 6B) will illustrate the number of repetitions that can be cycled during that set or series of exercises. Keep in mind that exercises repeated more than eight repetitions become more endurance productive. Five to six repetitions are speed-strength productive, and three to four repetitions develop more explosive strength. If one to two repetitions are the maximum, usually the exercises are executed with a high and heavy percentile weight. The most productive number of repetitions for speed-strength (mass) is five to six.

TABLE 6A

Speed-Strength Training Zones

Zone	Percentage	Weight Zone	Category
1st Zone	Less than 60%	Light wt. zone	SMALL
2nd Zone	60% - 69%	Light Heavy wt. zone	SMALL
3rd Zone	70% - 79%	Medium wt. zone	MEDIUM
4th Zone	80 - 89%	Heavy wt. zone	MEDIUM
5th Zone	90% - 99%	Super Heavy wt. zone	BIG
6th Zone	100% and plus +	Max wt.	

TABLE 6B

Classification of the Athlete	Example of One Exercise and the Number of Repetitions to Be Done in the Training Session	Volume = Maximum Repetitions Per Exercise
Beginner	$\frac{50}{5}$ $\frac{60}{5}$ 2 = total 15 reps	14-20
Intermediate	$\frac{50}{5}$ $\frac{60}{4}$ 2 $\frac{70}{4}$ $\frac{75}{4}$ 2 = total 25 reps	21-25
Advanced	$\frac{50}{5}$ 2 $\frac{60}{5}$ $\frac{70}{4}$ 2 $\frac{80}{3}$ 2 = total 29 reps	26-30
Elite	$\frac{50}{5}$ $\frac{60}{4}$ 2 $\frac{70}{3}$ 2 $\frac{75}{3}$ 4 $\frac{85}{1}$ 3 = total 34 reps	31-36

Reps = Repetitions

STEP 4: INTENSITY

The football coach is aware of the intensity (the amount of weight being lifted) which determines how strong the athlete is and what exercise movements are within his limits of correct performance. Only after initial testing and supervision should the athlete be allowed to perform movements in the high percentile ranges of weight. The information collected during initial testing and post-testing allows for new personal records (PRs) and new absolute speed-strength (one repetition maximum). The example used in the preparatory phase of the power snatch reads $\frac{50}{5}$ $\frac{55}{5}$ $\frac{60}{5}$ 2. These three sets of numbers show the 5-5-5/ volume levels of these three sets: (1) 50 percent of the 5 repetition maximum in the power snatch, (2) 55 percent of the 5 repetition maximum in the power snatch and (3) 60 percent of the 5 repetition maximum in the power snatch for two sets. By using the percentage chart (Chart 2, see page 25), the example of the power snatch shows that this athlete can lift 135 pounds in the power snatch for a one repetition maximum lift that had been a previous personal record. His goal is 150 pounds, and this is the number that will be looked up on the chart. The chart reads 50 percent of 150 pounds is 75 pounds for five repetitions, 55 percent of 150 pounds is 80 pounds and 60 percent of 155 pounds is 90 pounds for two sets of five repetitions. The challenge of the coach is to be well-versed concerning the intensity and number of repetitions needed which correlate correctly for that particular percentage of weight in relation to the number of repetitions (volume) that is used.

STEP 5: FREQUENCY OF WORKOUTS

Anything that is good can be overdone. That is what can happen when the speed-strength program is not planned and carried out properly. During the preparatory phase, the use of four lifting days is excellent during that football program. Coaches can see a better distribution of exercises and better use of the developing athlete's time. Some coaches still adhere to a three-day lifting schedule, but the four-day schedule has a greater advantage because of the volume and intensity of exercises that can be duplicated from workout to workout. In the competitive phase, the least amount of workouts should not be below two or more than four as a maximum. Remember that the frequency of workouts is also held in check by the volume (number of repetitions that can be performed per exercise).

Combinations of workout days are left to the discretion of the coach or trainer. Each team has a different personality; it is up to the coach to know what will best prepare his football team. Possible schedules of frequency of workouts in the preparatory phase are shown below:

4-DAY	**4-DAY**	**3-DAY**	**3-DAY**
Monday	Monday	Monday	Monday
Tuesday	Tuesday	Wednesday	Tuesday
Thursday	Wednesday	Friday	Friday
Friday	Friday		

An example of frequency of workouts in the main-competitive period is illustrated below:

4-DAY	**3-DAY**	**3-DAY**
Saturday	Saturday	Sunday
Monday	Monday	Monday
Tuesday	Wednesday	Wednesday
Wednesday		

In the preparatory phase, some coaches do use Saturdays during the summer and winter months to train. During the competitive phase, one must keep in mind the time during which the speed-strength training program is incorporated. Note that certain days have longer practices than others.

STEP 6: WARM-UP ROUTINE

The days of having an athlete just walk into the weight room and start lifting should be over. For example, the safety of the athlete is a top priority and the warm-up routine minimizes injury due to carelessness. The warm-up routine is a safeguard against the lack of preparation before starting the speed-strength program.

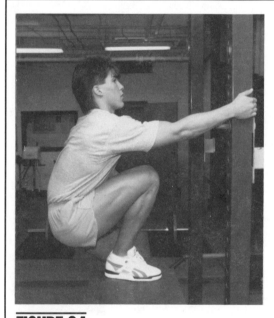

FIGURE 24

One-legged Squat

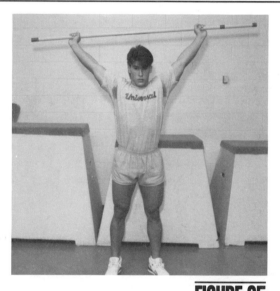

FIGURE 25

Upper Shoulder Flexors

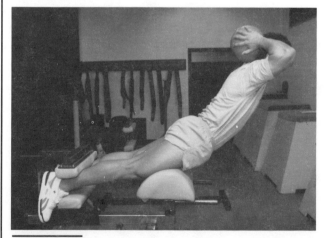

FIGURE 26

Glute Ham raises

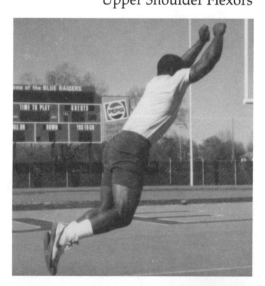

FIGURE 27

Long Jumps

EXERCISE CHART 2

Repetition Poundage Chart to Determine Load - In Increments of 5

ONE REPETITION MAXIMUM	50%	55%	60%	65%	70%	75%	80%	85%	90%	95%
600	300	330	360	390	420	450	480	510	540	570
595	300	325	355	385	415	445	475	505	535	565
590	295	325	355	385	415	440	470	500	530	560
585	290	320	350	380	410	440	470	495	525	555
580	290	320	350	375	405	435	465	495	520	550
575	290	315	345	375	400	430	460	490	520	545
570	285	315	340	370	400	430	455	485	515	540
565	280	310	340	365	395	425	450	480	510	535
560	280	310	335	365	390	420	450	475	505	530
555	280	305	335	360	390	415	445	470	500	525
550	275	300	330	360	385	410	440	470	495	520
545	270	300	325	355	380	410	435	465	490	520
540	270	295	325	350	380	405	430	460	485	515
535	270	295	320	350	375	400	430	455	480	510
530	265	290	320	345	370	400	425	450	475	505
525	260	290	315	340	370	395	420	445	470	500
520	260	285	310	340	365	390	415	440	470	495
515	260	285	310	335	360	385	410	440	465	490
510	255	280	305	330	355	380	410	435	460	485
505	250	280	305	330	355	380	405	430	455	480
500	250	275	300	325	350	375	400	425	450	475
495	250	270	295	320	345	370	395	420	445	470
490	245	270	295	320	345	370	390	415	440	465
485	240	265	290	315	340	365	390	410	435	460
480	240	265	290	310	335	360	385	410	430	455
475	240	260	285	310	330	355	380	405	430	450
470	235	260	280	305	330	350	375	400	425	445
465	230	255	280	300	325	350	370	395	420	440
460	230	255	275	300	320	345	370	390	415	435
455	230	250	275	295	320	340	365	385	410	430
450	225	250	270	290	315	340	360	380	405	430
445	220	245	265	290	310	335	355	380	400	425
440	220	240	265	285	310	330	350	375	395	420
435	220	240	260	285	305	325	350	370	390	415
430	215	235	260	280	300	320	345	365	385	410
425	210	235	255	275	300	320	340	360	380	405
420	210	230	250	275	295	315	335	355	380	400
415	210	230	250	270	290	310	330	355	375	395
410	205	225	245	265	285	310	330	350	370	390
405	200	225	245	265	285	305	325	345	365	385
400	200	220	240	260	280	300	320	340	360	380
395	200	215	235	255	275	295	315	335	355	375
390	195	215	235	255	275	290	310	330	350	370
385	190	210	230	250	270	290	310	325	345	365
380	190	210	230	245	265	285	305	325	340	360
375	190	205	225	245	260	280	300	320	340	355
370	185	205	220	240	260	280	295	315	335	350
365	180	200	220	235	255	275	290	310	330	345
360	180	200	215	235	250	270	290	305	325	340
355	180	195	215	230	250	265	285	300	320	335
350	175	190	210	230	245	260	280	300	315	330
345	170	190	205	225	240	260	275	295	310	330
340	170	185	205	220	240	255	270	290	305	325
335	170	185	200	220	235	250	270	285	300	320
330	165	180	200	215	230	250	265	280	295	315
325	160	180	195	210	230	245	260	275	290	310
320	160	175	190	210	225	240	255	270	290	305
315	160	175	190	205	220	235	250	270	285	300
310	155	170	185	200	215	230	250	265	280	295
305	150	170	185	200	215	230	245	260	275	290
300	150	165	180	195	210	225	240	255	270	285
295	150	160	175	190	205	220	235	250	265	280
290	145	160	175	190	205	220	230	245	260	275
285	140	155	170	185	200	215	230	240	255	270
280	140	155	170	180	195	210	225	240	250	265
275	140	150	165	180	190	205	220	235	250	260
270	135	150	160	175	190	200	215	230	245	255
265	130	145	160	170	185	200	210	225	240	250
260	130	145	155	170	180	195	210	220	235	245
255	130	140	155	165	180	190	205	215	230	240
250	125	140	150	160	175	190	200	210	225	240
245	120	135	145	160	170	185	195	210	220	235
240	120	130	145	155	170	180	190	205	215	230
235	120	130	140	155	165	175	190	200	210	225
230	115	125	140	150	160	170	185	195	205	220
225	110	125	135	145	160	170	180	190	200	215
220	110	120	130	145	155	165	175	185	200	210
215	110	120	130	140	150	160	170	185	195	205
210	105	115	125	135	145	160	170	180	190	200
205	100	115	125	135	145	155	165	175	185	195
200	100	110	120	130	140	150	160	170	180	190
195	100	105	115	125	135	145	155	165	175	185
190	95	105	115	125	135	140	150	160	170	180
185	90	100	110	120	130	140	150	155	165	175
180	90	100	110	115	125	135	145	155	160	170
175	90	95	105	115	120	130	140	150	160	165
170	85	95	100	110	120	130	135	145	155	160
165	80	90	100	105	115	125	130	140	150	155
160	80	90	95	105	110	120	130	135	145	150
155	80	85	95	100	110	115	125	130	140	145
150	75	80	90	100	105	110	120	130	135	140
145	70	80	85	95	100	110	115	125	130	140
140	70	75	85	90	100	105	110	120	125	135
135	70	75	80	90	95	100	110	115	120	130
130	65	70	80	85	90	100	105	110	115	125
125	60	70	75	80	90	95	100	105	110	120
120	60	65	70	80	85	90	95	100	110	115
115	60	65	70	75	80	85	90	100	105	110
110	55	60	65	70	75	80	90	95	100	105
105	50	60	65	70	75	80	85	90	95	100
100	50	55	60	65	70	75	80	85	90	95

Repetition Poundage Chart to Determine Load - In Increments of 10

ONE REPETITION MAXIMUM	50%	55%	60%	65%	70%	75%	80%	85%	90%	95%
600	300	330	360	390	420	450	480	510	540	570
590	295	325	355	385	415	440	470	500	530	560
580	290	320	350	375	405	435	465	495	520	550
570	285	315	340	370	400	430	455	485	515	540
560	280	310	335	365	390	420	450	475	505	530
550	275	300	330	360	385	410	440	470	495	520
540	270	295	325	350	380	405	430	460	485	515
530	265	290	320	345	370	400	425	450	475	505
520	260	285	310	340	365	390	415	440	470	495
510	255	280	305	330	355	380	410	435	460	485
500	250	275	300	325	350	375	400	425	450	475
490	245	270	295	320	345	370	390	415	440	465
480	240	265	290	310	335	360	385	410	430	455
470	235	260	280	305	330	350	375	400	425	445
460	230	255	275	300	320	345	370	390	415	435
450	225	250	270	290	315	340	360	380	405	430
440	220	240	265	285	310	330	350	375	395	420
430	215	235	260	280	300	320	345	365	385	410
420	210	230	250	275	295	315	335	355	380	400
410	205	225	245	265	285	310	330	350	370	390
400	200	220	240	260	280	300	320	340	360	380
390	195	215	235	255	275	290	310	330	350	370
380	190	210	230	245	265	285	305	325	340	360
370	185	205	220	240	260	280	295	315	335	350
360	180	200	215	235	250	270	290	305	325	340
350	175	190	210	230	245	260	280	300	315	330
340	170	185	205	220	240	255	270	290	305	325
330	165	180	200	215	230	250	265	280	295	315
320	160	175	190	210	225	240	255	270	290	305
310	155	170	185	200	215	230	250	265	280	295
300	150	165	180	195	210	220	240	255	270	285
290	145	160	175	190	205	220	230	245	260	275
280	140	155	170	180	195	210	225	240	250	265
270	135	150	160	175	190	200	215	230	245	255
260	130	145	155	170	180	195	210	220	235	245
250	125	140	150	160	175	190	200	210	225	240
240	120	130	145	155	170	180	190	205	215	230
230	115	125	140	150	160	170	185	195	205	220
220	110	120	130	145	155	165	175	185	200	210
210	105	115	125	135	145	160	170	180	190	200
200	100	110	120	130	140	150	160	170	180	190
190	95	105	115	125	135	140	150	160	170	180
180	90	100	110	115	125	135	145	155	160	170
170	85	95	100	110	120	130	135	145	155	160
160	80	90	95	105	110	120	130	135	145	150
150	75	80	90	100	105	110	120	130	135	140
140	70	75	85	90	100	105	110	120	125	135
130	65	70	80	85	90	100	105	110	115	125
120	60	65	70	80	85	90	95	100	110	115
110	55	60	65	70	75	80	90	95	100	105
100	50	55	60	65	70	75	80	85	90	95

The preparatory phase warm-up routine should read:

Warm-up routine
1. Jog 440 yards, medium speed
2. One-legged squat--3 sets x 8 repetitions (Figure 24)
3. Upper shoulder flexors--3 sets x 8 repetitions (Figure 25)
4. Glute ham raises--3 sets x 8 repetitions (Figure 26)
5. Ten long jumps or ten vertical jumps (Figure 27)

The 440-yard jog is done any time the athletes have not been running before they enter the weight room.

As in the competitive phase, if an athlete lifts after practice, the 440-yard jog would not be necessary. In the transitional phase, the warm-up is similar to the preparatory, except that the number of sets is changed to two sets instead of three sets.

STEP 7: RELAXATION AND FLEXIBILITY ROUTINE

Regardless of the training phase, the coach should implement the relaxation and flexibility routine (warm-down). This aspect of the speed-strength training program helps in the athlete's recovery and restoration from football practice or conditioning practice in the preparatory phase. Mental fatigue and soreness are remedied, and physical conditioning can be improved

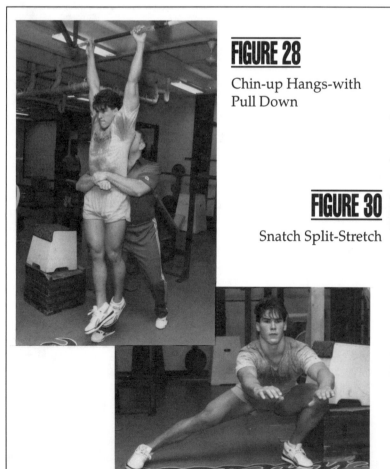

FIGURE 28

Chin-up Hangs-with Pull Down

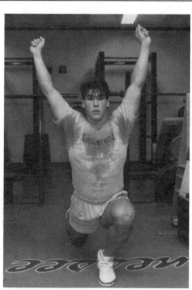

FIGURE 30

Snatch Split-Stretch

FIGURE 29

Side-to-side Stretch

by incorporating a relaxation and flexibility routine at the end of each workout. An example of the preparatory phase for relaxation and flexibility routine is shown below:

1. Chin-up hangs--with pull down, 3 sets x 6 seconds (Figure 28)
2. Side to side--stretch, 3 sets x 8 repetitions (Figure 29)
3. Snatch split--stretch--3 sets x 8 repetitions (Figure 30)
4. Russian shower--before leaving the shower, gradually turn the cold water up and turn the hot water off. Using the cold water shower is a way to message and stimulate the body, particularly in areas that have experienced trauma or injury and feel like they will be sore. Use a five to ten minute time zone.

STEP 8: VARIABILITY OF THE LOAD

According to Coach Goldstein, the training loads must be varied, simply because of how quickly the athlete's body adapts to a specific movement and specific exercise.

The use of percentages and repetitions (Table 7) will help the coach adjust the training program to properly progress to the percentage and repetition levels. By understanding the big, medium, and small percentages, coaches' athletes are less likely to fail to progress.

TABLE 7
Speed-Strength Training Repetitions
Percentages and Repetitions

Exercises	40-49%	50-59%	60-69%	70-79%	80-89%	90-100%
Squats	5-8	5-8	3-6	1-5	1-4	1-2
Snatchs	5-8	4-6	2-5	1-5	1-3	1-2
Cleans	5-8	4-6	2-5	1-5	1-4	1-2
Good Mornings	5-8	4-6	3-5	2-5	2-4	1-2
Presses	5-8	3-6	2-5	1-5	1-4	1-2
Jerks	5-8	3-6	2-5	1-4	1-3	1-2

TABLE 8
Qualities of Speed-Strength Training

1-3 Rep's = Power growth will be larger but not in Mass of the athlete.

4-6 Rep's = Muscle Mass increase – growth of power will be lower.

7-10 Rep's = Muscle Mass and power will be lower. Endurance is greater.

An example of excellent planning is shown below:

Week 1   **2nd Workout with Power Clean**
Power Clean $\frac{50}{5}$ $\frac{60}{5}$ $\frac{65}{4}$ 2 $\frac{55}{5}$ $\frac{65}{4}$ $\frac{75}{3}$ $\frac{80}{2}$ 2

It is useful to know the correct qualities (Table 8) and then assign the correct percent in the speed-strength program exercises.

STEP 9: NUMBER OF EXERCISES

There should be a prescribed limit to the number of exercises in one training session. In the preparatory phase, the number of exercises would be no less than five and no more than eight. In an exercise, volume and intensity are cycled from small-medium-big which are derived from a maximum (absolute effort) number of lifting movements of speed-strength. Examples are: (1) power clean, (2) bench press, (3) back squat and (4) jerk from stand. A cycle of training can be derived from a maximum number of these exercises. Another example is that (nonspecific) general, plyometrics, ballistics, neck, abdominal and gymnastic movements are not included, but they are aspects of the total program. Total programming involves no less than eight and no more than fourteen speed-strength exercises. In the competitive phase, the speed-strength lifting movements would be no less than three and no more than five. The total speed-strength program would be no less than six and no more than ten. Note that in the pre-competitive period, the number can vary from one lift a day to three lifts a day, with one or two exercise (nonspecific) movements added. The amount of practice the athletes are subjected to should be constantly monitored by the coach.

SUMMARY

Following the nine steps for the implementation of a speed-strength training program will allow the football coach, trainer or athlete an opportunity to incorporate the four components of speed-strength, thus providing the key elements and foundation for a successful competitive edge for his football team and players.

CHECKPOINTS IN IMPLEMENTING A SPEED-STRENGTH TRAINING PROGRAM

1. **Periods** - time of annual plan (Pre-competitive, competitive and transitional)

2. **Task** - what exercise or exercises chosen (The main goal) What the coach wants during this period

3. **Preparation** - condition of the athlete (Consideration in planning the athletic program)

4. **Length of sport career** - high school time period (Ninth-twelfth grade)

5. **Age of athlete** - 15-18 years old (average ages)

6. **Body weight** - measure of body weight

7. **Training loads** - amount of volume + intensity recorded (Records and charts)

8. **Volume of the program** - number of reps used per exercise per day

9. **Intensity** - amount of weight being used

10. **Quality and character of the exercise** - kind of movement skill being used

11. **Character of exercise**
    A. For speed
    B. For strength
    C. For flexibility, etc.

12. **Loading** - what reps and weight is being used in training cycle

13. **Order** - order of exercise and arrangement—speed to strength

14. **Tempo** - execution of speed-strength in the exercise movement

15. **Volume + intensity of training period** - having a plan—daily, weekly, monthly, yearly

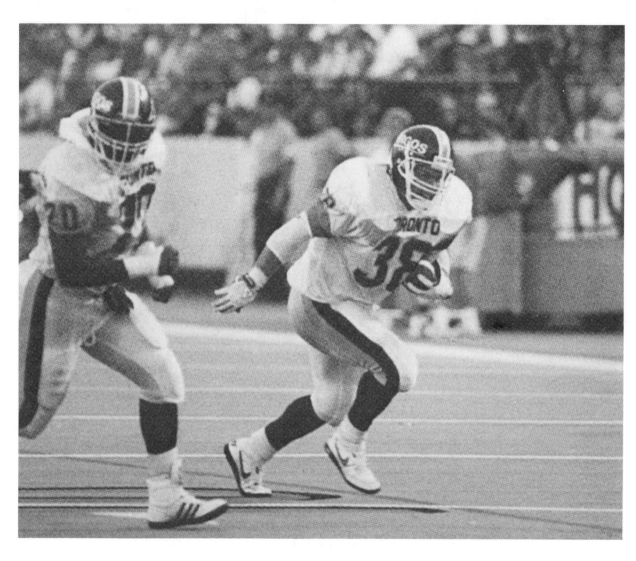

"Speed-strength training for football is about building the best football body."
E.J. "Doc" Kreis

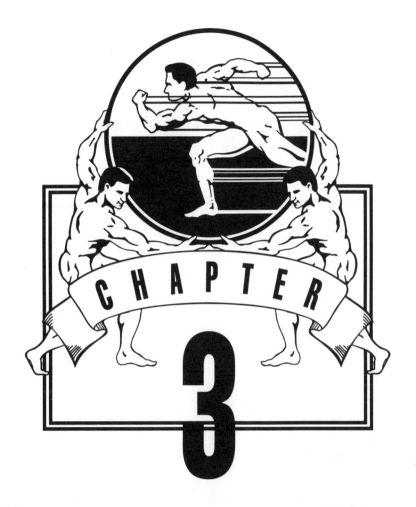

SNATCH AND CLEAN EXERCISES

"If people knew how hard I have had to work to gain my mastery, it wouldn't seem wonderful at all."

Michelangelo
Italian Painter/Sculptor

SNATCH AND CLEAN EXERCISES

There is not a football coach anywhere who does not want to find an athlete with potential talent and skill and start him on the pathway to college and professional ranks. To do this, much depends on which training principles the football coach will rely on during this formative time. In working with the football player, proper selection of lifting exercises is an essential key to the success or failure in development of speed-strength. This chapter describes the snatch and clean lifting exercises and discusses starting positions and grips, action of the lifts and coaching tips. These lifting exercises are designed to enhance the athlete's speed-strength development. Additional information on full-range movement is also discussed.

LIFTING EXERCISES--FULL-RANGE MOVEMENTS

Speed-strength lifting exercises should emphasize a full range of movements. Full-range movements build more strength in the muscles, tendons and ligaments because more muscle fibers become involved in the exercise movement.

THE STARTING POSITION AND GRIPS

The initial movement of all lifting exercises from the floor is referred to as the starting position. It is also the position in which the coach will instruct players to return to when completing each exercise. The main points of the starting position include:

1. Feet--hip-width apart with the weight of the body evenly distributed over the base from toe to heel--the insteps are underneath the bar so that you are close to it

2. Knees--bent to approximately 90 degrees with the seat a little higher than the knee joint

3. Back--maintained in a flat, strong position--remember that "flat" can be at any angle and does not mean vertical

4. Hands--positioned to give the desired leverage and keeping the arms straight

5. Shoulders--above and slightly in front of the barbell

6. Head--in a comfortable position with the eyes looking slightly up

With dynamic position, resistance of the barbell is overcome by the major muscles of the legs and hips while maintaining the back in the Universal Athlete Position.

THE GRIPS

The position taken while holding the bar or grip should be taught from the very beginning. The standard grip is the hook style. In the hook grip, the thumb is placed under the bar with the fingers placed firmly over the top. After learning this basic grip, the athlete can then learn to use the three widths of the grip, wide (near sleeves), medium (shoulder width) and narrow (toward the center). Grip-width in the snatch is very important. The greatest advantage of the wide grip is the ability of the athlete to retain his position under the bar. The use of the medium grip is more prevalent in the pressing, pushing and cleaning exercises. The use of the narrow grip is more distinct in the specialty movements of an exercise and in certain specialty situations that may call for using a narrow grip.

SNATCH EXERCISES

The snatch exercise is one of the two classical Olympic lifts, the other being the clean and jerk. The snatch is the lifting movement of the bar overhead onto straight arms in one movement. The two-hand snatch is performed in an uninterrupted movement of the bar from the floor to a fully-straight arm position overhead. The snatch is the fastest and most explosive movement.

The snatch has three consecutively performed parts: (1) starting position (Figure 31), (2) the lift upward to full extension (Figure 32), and (3) the drop under the bar (Figure 33) and recovery to standing position (Figure 34).

There are four different styles of performing the snatch exercises: (1) power snatch, (2) the split, (3) muscle, (4) the squat style or Olympic style. Each style has two starting positions: (1) the static start, which is also called the start without preparatory movement, and (2) the dynamic start. The static start is rarely used because of the technique and method of tearing or ripping the barbell from the platform instead of lifting. The most widely used start is the dynamic start. The majority of football players should adopt a variation of the dynamic start. First, the knee and ankle joints are in line. The second part before the lifting of the bar from the platform is the stage of raising the hips, increasing the angles of the knee and ankle joints.

This position taken in the preparatory action the moment the bar breaks from the platform is called the dynamic start.

POWER SNATCH-EXERCISE 1

STARTING POSITION

From the basic stance or starting position, the hands are positioned on the barbell using the wide grip-width.

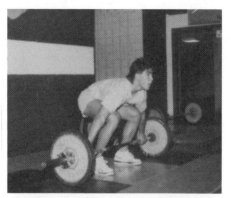

FIGURE 31

Starting position in the snatch

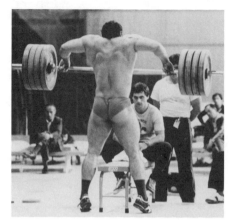

FIGURE 32

The Lift to full Extension

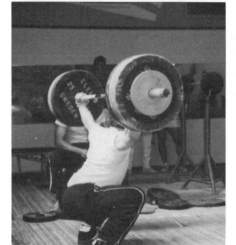

FIGURE 33

The Drop Under the Bar

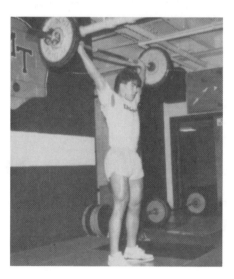

FIGURE 34

Recovery to Standing Position

THE ACTION LIFT

The upward pull is initiated when the barbell leaves the floor past the upper thighs and with extension through the hips and toes in preparation of dropping under the bar. The bar will be almost above the waist.

The drive to lock-out (Figure 35) continues at the same time forcing the hips in and upwards, while pulling strongly with the arms and shoulders until final extension is locked in with the high squat finish of the feet and bar in the overhead position. The power snatch final position is not as low as the squat style snatch. This exercise will be more in line with what athletes will master in form, method and technique.

SPEED-STRENGTH COACHING TIPS

This is a great movement of exercise for speed development and strength. Check to make sure the athlete is balanced on his feet from toe to heel in the "starting position." Remember that this is a dynamic starting motion that can have great benefits for transfer to the football field. The power snatch is an excellent explosive strength movement.

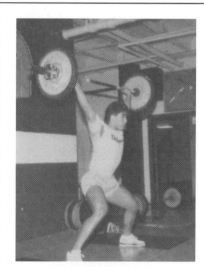

FIGURE 35

Power Snatch Position of Lock-out

SPLIT SNATCH-EXERCISE 2

STARTING POSITION

Repeat the correct starting position stance as used in the power snatch. Hands are positioned in the wide-grip width.

THE ACTION OF THE LIFT

This action is the same as in the power snatch when the first movement onto the toes is completed as the bar is about the level of the tops of the thighs.

It is essential to carry out the lift of the bar to the level of the waist with the balance pivoted on both feet. But, beginning at this level in the split style, the lifter moves his center of gravity onto that leg, which is to be moved forward half a step. But the other leg must travel significantly further, about two to three times further. Therefore, the lifter maintains his balance on one leg, while the other leg is being moved backwards, by not more than one-third or half-way.

The position of the bar is still continuing to move upwards by the action of the arm and shoulder muscles. From this point of the split extension, the recovery is achieved by extending the forward leg and then the other (back) leg. The distance that the bar is pulled in the split snatch is much higher than the power snatch. The additional distance that the bar must travel makes the split style excellent for training to develop more coordination and quick-feet movement (Figure 36). It also helps the young ball player develop hip and leg flexibility and balance agility in an athletic motion. The additional height that occurs from the pull makes for more and faster muscle use being coordinated into the pulling. The split snatch is an excellent explosive exercise.

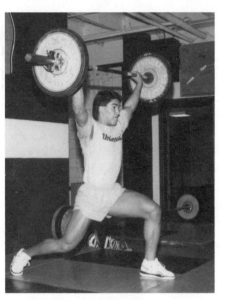

FIGURE 36

Split Snatch Position

MUSCLE SNATCH--EXERCISE 3

STARTING POSITION

Repeat the correct starting position stance as used in the power snatch. Hands are positioned in the wide grip-width.

THE ACTION OF THE LIFT

The action of the lift is the same as in the power snatch. The only difference is there should be very little or no flexion of the knees--as if trying to keep the hips and legs from dropping at all (Figure 37).

SPEED-STRENGTH COACHING TIPS

The muscle snatch is just what its name represents--muscle. The degree of flexion increases the more the muscle is used in completing the muscle snatch. The amount of weight will be less than is used in the split snatch and power snatch.

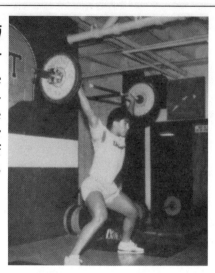

FIGURE 37

Muscle Snatch - Should have very little or no Flexion of the Knees

OLYMPIC STYLE SNATCH (SQUAT SNATCH)-EXERCISE 4

STARTING POSITION

Repeat the correct starting position stance as used in previous snatch style lifts. Hands are positioned in the wide grip-width.

THE ACTION OF THE LIFT

This is the same as in the power snatch, the only difference being the squat position under the bar--putting the athlete in a low squat stance with the bar locked overhead (Figure 38).

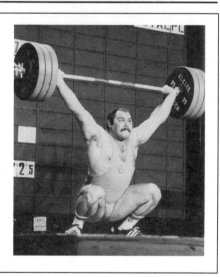

FIGURE 38

Olympic Style Snatch

SPEED-STRENGTH COACHING TIPS

This is one of the classic Olympic lifts. The athlete who masters the form, method and technique will have tremendous coordination and dexterity. *This is the ultimate in the snatch style exercises.*

SNATCH PULL - EXERCISE 5

STARTING POSITION

Repeat the correct starting position stance as used in previous snatch style lifts. Hands are positioned in the wide grip-width.

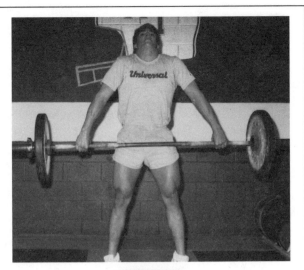

FIGURE 39

Snatch Pull in the final Stage of the Pull

THE ACTION OF THE LIFT

This is the same as in the other snatch exercises, except the movement is only taken to the point right past the top of the thighs or right above the groin. After the forcing of the hips in and upwards, the bar is returned to the floor. The arms and shoulders rise upward to pinch at the base of the neck, utilizing the trapezius muscles in the finishing pull (Figure 39).

SPEED-STRENGTH COACHING TIPS

The amount of weight will be much higher then that used in the power, split, muscle and Olympic styles. The use of lifting straps can aid when more additional weight is used in performing this movement. Remember to let the grip stay wide and to pinch the arms to the shoulders and shoulders to the neck.

HANG SNATCH-EXERCISE 6

STARTING POSITION.

From the starting position, the hands should be placed in the wide-grip position and the correct starting position either from the hang (standing erect barbell and hanging) or from designated heights (boxes or racks) (Figure 40).

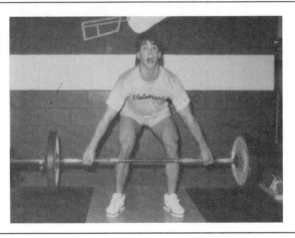

FIGURE 40

Hang Snatch Starting

PULLING MOVEMENT

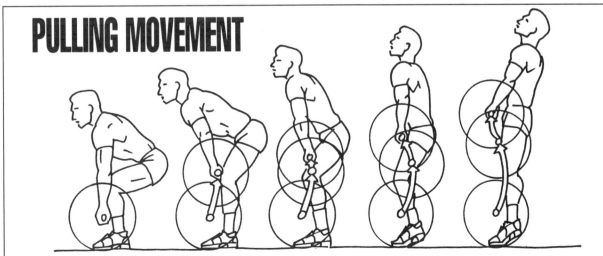

POSITION WITH BARBELL HANGING
THE ACTION OF THE LIFT

The action of the hang snatch begins with the bar resting at mid-thigh level and straight-arm position. This is where the expression "hang" comes from. The method and technique of completing the hang snatch are mechanical, the same as in the power split, muscle and Olympic styles.

SPEED-STRENGTH COACHING TIPS

This would be a good movement to do as the last snatch lift before resting prior to a Friday football game. It involves less work on the back and is extremely explosive. The hang snatch also can be used easily from the blocks or racks.

ONE-ARM DUMBBELL SNATCH-EXERCISE 7
STARTING POSITION

The feet are a little more than shoulder-width apart, with the toes turned outward slightly. The dumbbell is positioned between the athlete's two legs on the floor; take a squat-like position over the dumbbell. Let's start with the right hand, gripping the dumbbell and the left in a balancing position on the left thigh.

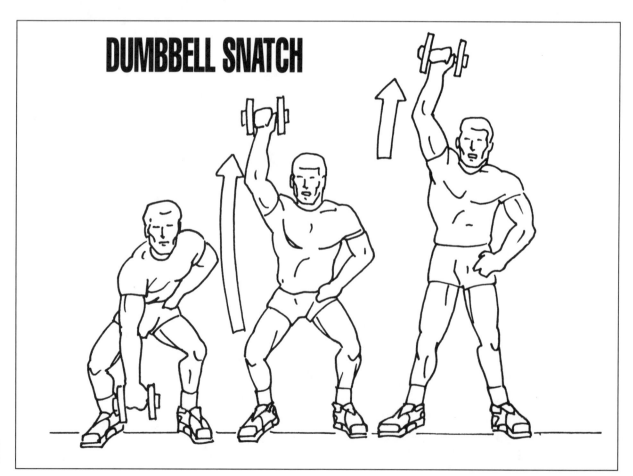

DUMBBELL SNATCH

THE ACTION OF THE LIFT

The dumbbell is then pulled in an upward movement and driven back-up. The hip and shoulder muscles continue to support the dumbbell until the desired extension is obtained.
Once the number of repetitions is completed with one arm, then switch and repeat with the other arm. The dynamic starting movement requires that the free arm (not holding the dumbbell) act as a balancing aid in the successful completion of the lift.

SPEED-STRENGTH COACHING TIPS

This is an excellent lift to be used in preparation for an athletic event. It involves less work from the lower back, and the demand is less a factor in fatiguing the athlete.

SNATCH PULL-HIGH PULL-EXERCISE 8

STARTING POSITION

As in the snatch-pull movement, the starting position is again repeated, using the wide grip hand position as customary in the snatch exercise.

THE ACTION OF THE LIFT

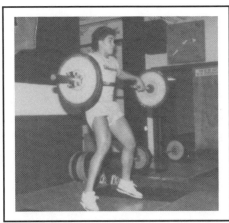

After the bar completes the first and second pull, the elbows will make the breaking pull from the waist to the chin of the athlete. Again, make the full extension of the hips to the toes raising to the top, allowing the completion of the lift. This is what makes the snatch pull-high pull different from the snatch and snatch pull (See picture).

SPEED-STRENGTH COACHING TIPS

The amount of weight will be lighter than weight used in the snatch pull exercise because of the elbow-breaking movement.

Remind the athlete to drive with the hips to the tip of his toes. This is a super exercise for lower and upper back development and coordination for sports transfer.

CLEAN EXERCISE

The clean exercise is just the first half of the Olympic classical lift, the clean and jerk. Again, the position used is basic to all pulling exercises and to all movements when the weight is lifted from the floor. It will also be the position to which the athlete will return when the lift is completed. The principles that apply to the snatch also apply to the clean. The difference is medium-grip and finishing movement. This position provides for the additional level of strength that can be exerted using this style. *Strength Coach Bill Starr calls the clean the athlete's exercise simply because of the amount of speed used from start to finish.*

POWER CLEAN-EXERCISE 1

STARTING POSITION

The starting position is the same as in the snatch lifts. The feet will be a little wider and the grip is the medium-grip (Figure 41).

THE ACTION OF THE LIFT

The position of the athlete is the same as in the snatch movement, except for the grip position. The difference in movements is that the clean is stopped once the body has moved under the bar with the elbows pointing up and the weight resting on the pectoral and frontal deltoid muscles. It is important that the proper steps for completion of the lift and return to the floor be carried out as follows:

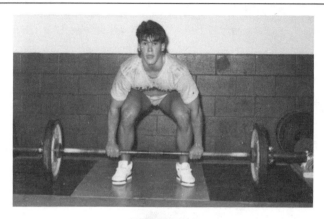

FIGURE 41

Power Clean Starting Position

1. The starting position and the pull off the floor should be an easy strong pull;

2. The second pull (starts from right above the knees) is where the explosive speed is generated to force the hip and leg punch through the trunk (Figure 42). About the same time, the extension of the arms is locked by the follow-through of the shoulders, and in a "chair reaction," the clean is completed. As in the power snatch, the power clean will be in the squat style or Olympic style clean (Figure 43).

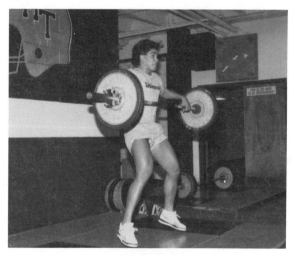

FIGURE 42

Power Clean Second Pull - Punching the Knees Forward

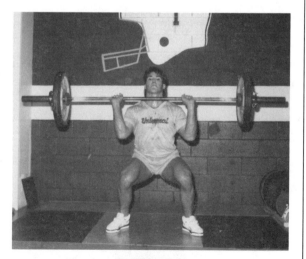

FIGURE 43

Power Clean After the Second Pull and the Drop is complete

SPEED-STRENGTH COACHING TIPS

"If your program only allowed you to do one exercise, this would be the best" (Starr). Examples of the motion of the power clean are when players are coming off the line of scrimmage in the execution of blocking and tackling. When teaching this movement, make sure the bar is kept close to the body in order to achieve maximum performance. Speed is the factor of the power clean that is important.

SPLIT CLEAN-EXERCISE 2

STARTING POSITION

The athlete is to repeat the same starting position as in the power clean, using the medium grip.

THE ACTION OF THE LIFT

As in the split snatch, the difference will be in leg position and not having to lift the bar past the chest and into the drop. Once the second pull is started, the center of gravity shifts onto that leg which is to be moved forward. The distance of the other leg will vary from the center of the starting position. Again, balance and coordination become key factors in completing the split clean exercise (Figure 44).

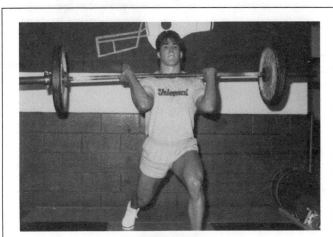

FIGURE 44

Split Clean - After the drop

SPEED-STRENGTH COACHING TIPS

The split clean is a difficult movement to teach because of the split method and technique. The athlete must exert more force because the additional height the bar must be pulled compared to the power and squat style clean. Follow the down movement of the bar in correct fashion back onto the floor.

MUSCLE CLEAN-EXERCISE 3

STARTING POSITION

Repeat the starting clean position of previous clean exercise lifts using the medium grip.

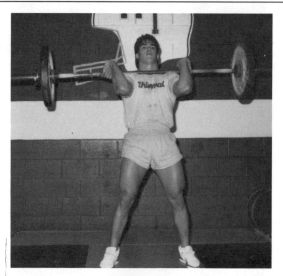

FIGURE 45

Muscle clean - has little or no Flexion of the Knees

THE ACTION OF THE LIFT

As in the muscle snatch, the flexion is little or none--as if trying (which the athlete is) not to bend or drop the hips and legs (Figure 45).

SPEED-STRENGTH COACHING TIPS

The muscle clean is literally what the name represents--muscle. The amount of weight will be lighter due to the height to which the weight is being pulled.

OLYMPIC STYLE CLEAN (SQUAT CLEAN)-EXERCISE 4

STARTING POSITION

Repeat the starting position used in previous clean style lifts using the medium grip.

THE ACTION OF THE LIFT

The difference in the squat (Olympic) clean is the position in which the bar is caught. After the hips drop, the low position of the hips and torso makes the Olympic clean different from the power and other listed cleans because of this low position (Figure 46).

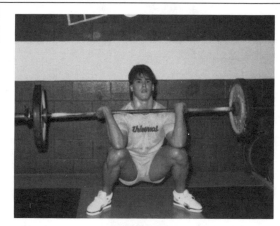

FIGURE 46

Olympic Style Clean

SPEED-STRENGTH COACHING TIPS

The two biggest mistakes made in the Olympic style clean are: (1) not keeping the back flat, which will hinder the amount of power that can be generated by the hip muscles and thighs and (2) trying to pull the weight off the floor with the arms, instead of using the arms as guide wires until the final pull. The success the athletes have will depend on the coordination of these movements into one explosive strength move.

CLEAN PULL--EXERCISE 5

STARTING POSITION

Repeat the correct starting position as in previous clean style lifts using medium grip.

THE ACTION OF THE LIFT

From the position of the second pull (along mid-thigh), the action of the lift is similar to the snatch pull exercise. Again, the extension to the drop position does <u>not</u> take place; the follow-through of the arms stays straight with the shoulders pinching the trapezius muscles to the neck (Figure 47).

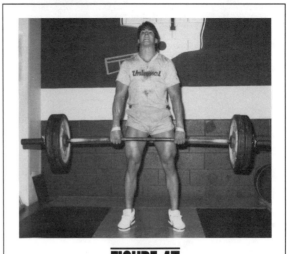

FIGURE 47

Clean Pull Action of the Lift - Weight Straps being worn

SPEED-STRENGTH COACHING TIPS

This is an excellent exercise for the overloading of weight, as well as to strengthen the pulling movements. The use of straps may also be of great benefit in helping the athlete maintain his grip in order to keep the bar from coming loose in his hands. Remember to remind your athletes not to bounce the weights off the platform. Use good form and good technique.

HANG CLEAN-EXERCISE 6

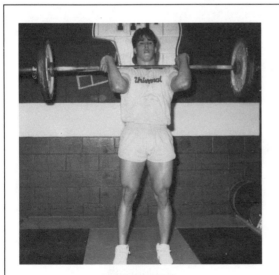

FIGURE 48

Elbows up in completing the Hang Clean

STARTING POSITION

The starting position is either with the athlete standing erect and the weight hanging or a standing position with the barbell in blocks or on the rack. (This may give the hang clean a different kind of starting point.) The medium grip is used (Figure 47).

THE ACTION OF THE LIFT

The position of the second pull is the starting point of the hang clean (bar hanging at mid-thigh). The movement used in making the clean from the second pull requires more back and hip leg movement because the weight is already in the second pull position. The movements from the second pull to the rack position are the same as in the power, split, muscle and Olympic cleans. Remember to have the athletes keep their elbows up (Figure 48).

SPEED-STRENGTH COACHING TIPS

The easiest way to learn the starting position would be to practice with the bar from the hang position. Learn the feel of the lift before attempting to put the total clean movement together.

DUMBBELL POWER CLEAN-EXERCISE 7

STARTING POSITION

Again, repeat the correct starting position stance as used in previous power clean exercise. Hands are positioned on the dumbbells to give the desired leverage and balance needed in coordinating the starting movement.

THE ACTION OF THE LIFT

The position of the athlete is the same as in the power clean movement except for the use of dumbbells rather than the barbell. Again, it is important to follow the proper steps for completion of the lift and return to the floor. Carry out as follows:

1. The starting position and the pull off the floor should be a strong, smooth pull.

2. The second pull (starts from just above the knees) is where the explosive speed is generated to force the hip and leg punch through the trunk and torso. About the same time, the extension of the arms is backed by the follow-through of the shoulders, and in a "chair reaction," the dumbbells are cleaned as in the power clean exercise (Figure 49).

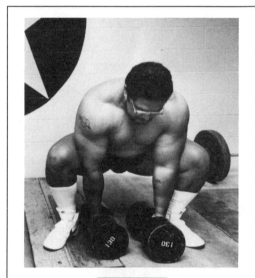

FIGURE 49

Dumbbell Power Clean

SPEED-STRENGTH COACHING TIPS

This is a tremendous exercise for teaching the athlete to raise through the hip to the toes and getting the full pulling motion. Also, the factors of balance, coordination and dexterity are invaluable to the overall development of the athlete. Again lifting straps can be used to allow the athlete to use more weight and maintain better control in the gripping of the dumbbell. Also, the beginning position is repeated with emphasis on keeping the chest out and shoulders back.

CLEAN PULL-HIGH PULL--EXERCISE 8

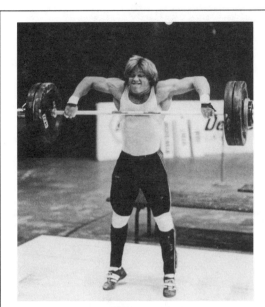

FIGURE 50

Clean Pull-High Pull

STARTING POSITION

Repeat the starting position used in the clean pull or power clean exercise. Using the medium grip, the second movement will result in the elbows bringing the Olympic bar to a high-pull position.

THE ACTION OF THE LIFT

After the bar completes the first and second pull and is moving into the finishing position in the clean pull, the additional part of this exercise is the high pull. Upon completion of the pull, the hips move in and upward as the bar is just above the groin; the elbows then are drawn up, which then allows the bar to travel to the position at the mid-chest. The arms and shoulders rise upward to pinch at the base of the neck, utilizing the back and trapezius muscle in the finishing pull (Figure 50).

SPEED-STRENGTH COACHING TIPS

The rising to the toes and the pulling of the bar to the chest will develop more body control. The use of lifting straps can aid in successfully completing this exercise because of the improved grip.

CLEAN AND JERK EXERCISE

The clean and jerk is the second lift of the Olympic classical lifts. It combines strength and speed into one exercise. For the football player, mastering the technique and method of this lift will pay off in the coordination of speed and strength. There are many carryovers from weight resistance training to the football field. The clean and jerk improves the feet coordination and the placement of the feet for recovery quickness.

CLEAN AND JERK (TWO-PART MOVEMENT)-EXERCISE 1

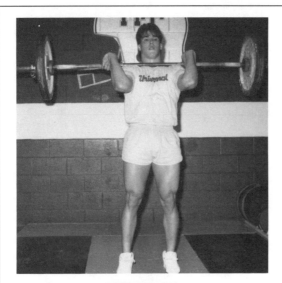

FIGURE 51

Clean and Jerk Starting Position into the Jerk

STARTING POSITION

Repeat the starting position used in the power clean. The second movement to the position is racking the bar across the chest and shoulders, as illustrated in the clean exercises (Figure 51). The medium grip is used.

THE ACTION OF THE LIFT

After completing the first clean phase of the clean and jerk, move to the second phase -- the completion of the jerk. As in the front press or military press (standing position), the back is straight with the elbows and head up. Dip the knees approximately six inches, and in one explosive jump, drive the weight overhead with the legs (Figure 52). The arms are used mainly as a guide for the weight, even though the athlete explosively presses with the arms as the entire body comes off the ground. The split movement will have one leg forward and one leg back--usually the dominant leg goes forward.

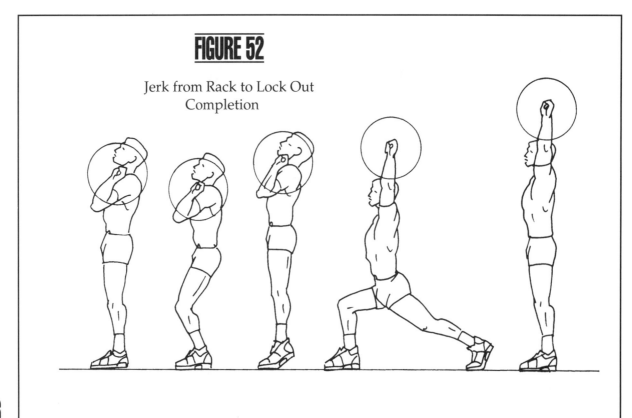

FIGURE 52

Jerk from Rack to Lock Out Completion

ACTION FOR JERK EXERCISE
(JERK BOX)

The Jerk Box shows the action of the feet from the start to the split movement of the Jerk

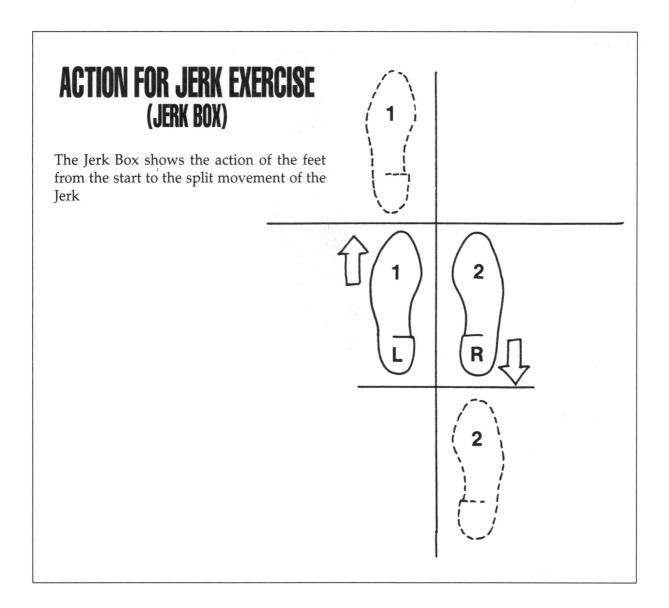

To return to an upright, erect position, push back with the front leg and begin to take the needed steps back to where both feet are hip-width apart and the barbell is supported overhead. Hold for a count of two seconds and upon completion, lower the bar to the starting position on the floor.

SPEED-STRENGTH COACHING TIPS

One mistake that is commonly made while performing the split movement of the jerk is stepping back with the back foot and not splitting the front foot forward. Splitting the feet and keeping the hips collected will keep the athlete positioned under the bar and also help in the development of explosiveness, balance and speed--the total qualities of speed-strength training.

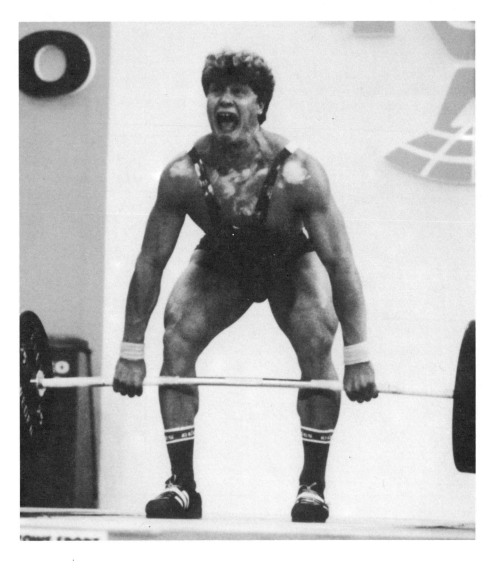

"Regardless of what strength is being used, there is no substitute for aggressive effort to success."
E. J. "Doc" Kreis

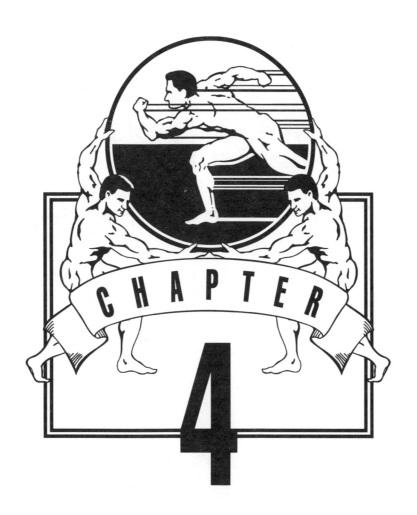

CHAPTER 4

PRESS EXERCISES

"Genius is one percent inspiration and ninety-nine percent perspiration. I never did anything worth doing by accident, nor did any of my inventions come by accident; they came by work."
Thomas Edison
American Inventor

PRESS EXERCISES

Because of football rules change, pressing exercises have become increasingly important. One of the most important rule changes has been the legal use of hands by offensive linemen. The importance of upper body strength, particularly in the chest, is more important than ever to the success of all football players. A strong upper body will allow the following hand positioning: (1) wide, (2) medium, and/or (3) narrow grip position, depending on the press exercise being used. Athletes should start with what is comfortable; then to obtain a wide hand position, move one hand width out. To obtain narrow grip position -- move one hand width in. The medium hand grip is comfortable for most athletes.

BENCH PRESS - EXERCISE 1

STARTING POSITION

Lie on the bench with the chest facing upward. The grip will vary from player to player.

THE ACTION OF THE LIFT

As the bar is removed from the rack or handed off to the lifter, the lifter lowers the barbell to the center of the chest at a point near the end of the sternum. This is more appropriately called the groove point or power zone. Then, touch the chest to again ensure a full-range of motion and extend the bar back in a quick, explosive motion (Figure 53).

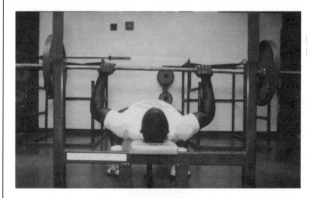

FIGURE 53

The Bench Press starting position

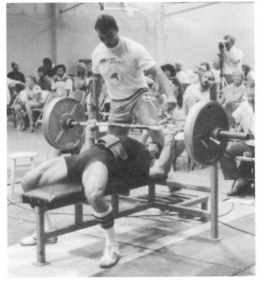

FIGURE 54

Bench Press - the Action of the Bar Moving Upward

This quick upward explosion builds speed-strength directly into the muscles, training the muscles to react quickly. Every exercise makes the muscles learn to react to this method. The transfer principle of exploding in the weight room will have the result of exploding power on the football field.

It is important to keep the hips and back on the bench throughout the exercise. That means no bridging. It is important to get the natural arch in order to allow the use of strength from the lattissimus muscles. The position of the feet provide the foundation of support on which the bench press force is generated. It is important once the foot position is in place that the feet stay firmly planted. As the bar is moving upward, the athlete should try to move it in a slight arch back over the eyes. The bar then does not move in a straight line, but from the center touch-down spot on the chest to the center of the head (Figure 54).

SPEED-STRENGTH COACHING TIPS

Make certain that the body is balanced and positioned on the bench before starting the lift. The use of spotters to aid and assist is a rule of the game. Having a big bench press is only important to the athletes if they transfer that strength to the football field. Do not over value a movement that is performed lying down.

INCLINE BENCH PRESS - EXERCISE 2

STARTING POSITION

Repeat the starting position that is used on the bench press. The angle of the bench indicates the proper foot position for maximum force using the medium grip (Figure 55).

THE ACTION OF THE LIFT

This involves lowering the position of the bar to the chest placed right under the chin. The action of returning to lock-out follows the same guidelines used in the bench press. Remember to push the bar slightly back as it is going up (Figure 56).

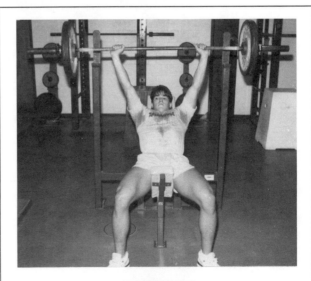

FIGURE 55

Incline Bench Press starting position

SPEED-STRENGTH COACHING TIPS

This is a good alternate exercise for football players because of the degree angle of the incline pressing motion.

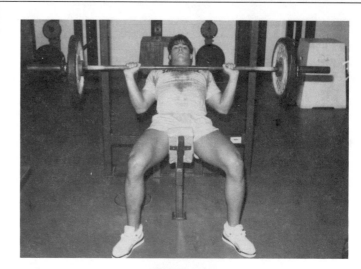

FIGURE 56

Bar at chest level and under chin

DUMBBELL BENCH PRESS - EXERCISE 3

STARTING POSITION

Repeat the starting position used in the barbell bench press. Because of the balancing factors of the two implements of weight, the feet may be a little farther apart than what is normally used in performing the barbell bench press. The grip depends on the balancing position of the dumbbell (Figure 57).

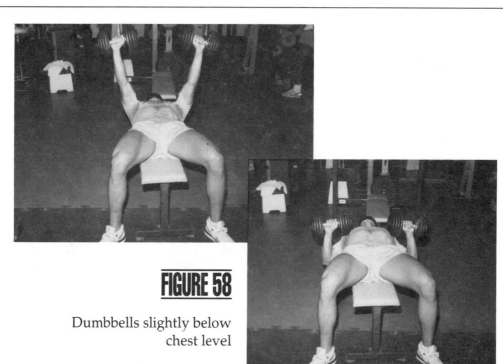

FIGURE 57

Dumbbell Bench Press starting position

FIGURE 58

Dumbbells slightly below chest level

THE ACTION OF THE LIFT

The dumbbells are lowered sideways from the starting position gradually, allowing the arms to torque to the position of the shoulder and armpit section. Upon making the full-range motion, return back to starting position (Figure 58).

SPEED STRENGTH COACHING TIPS

All dumbbell exercises require a great degree of control, and as a consequence, the muscle groups that are used in the movements have additional resistance placed upon them. Keep a watchful eye out for athletes having trouble controlling the exercise movement.

DUMBBELL INCLINE BENCH PRESS - EXERCISE 4

STARTING POSITION

Repeat the starting position as used in the dumbbell bench press (Figure 59). The grip depends on the balancing position.

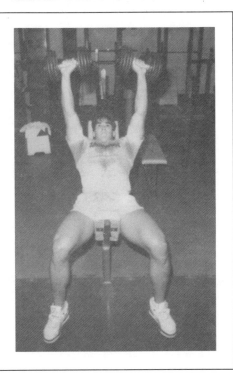

FIGURE 59

Dumbbell Incline Bench Press starting position

THE ACTION OF THE LIFT

The dumbbells are lowered sideways from the starting position, progressively allowing the arms to bend throughout the movement until the touching position is felt. Once the touch is made, the movement is then reversed and pressed back to the starting position (figure 60).

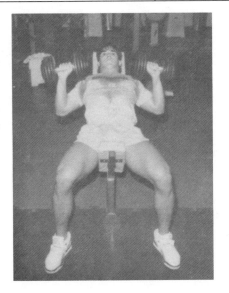

FIGURE 60

Dumbbells being lowered to chest level

SPEED STRENGTH COACHING TIPS

In using the dumbbell, as with a leverage movement, ease into the full-range movement through the initial repetitions. The lowering of the dumbbells should be controlled, and they should be brought back to the starting position in a dynamic fashion.

BEHIND THE NECK PRESS (STANDING) - EXERCISE 5

STARTING POSITION

The bar rests on the shoulders behind the neck. The grip position can be either the wide, medium or narrow. The feet are approximately hip-width apart (Figure 61)

THE ACTION OF THE LIFT

The barbell is pressed with dynamic force overhead to arms' length in a vertical line (Figure 62). Then lower the barbell back down into the starting position.

SPEED-STRENGTH COACHING TIPS

Before starting the lift, the body should be in a strong, well-braced and balanced position. The head is set slightly forward so the bar may travel in a vertical line from the shoulders. Note the lowering of the bar is done under control back to the starting position on the shoulders.

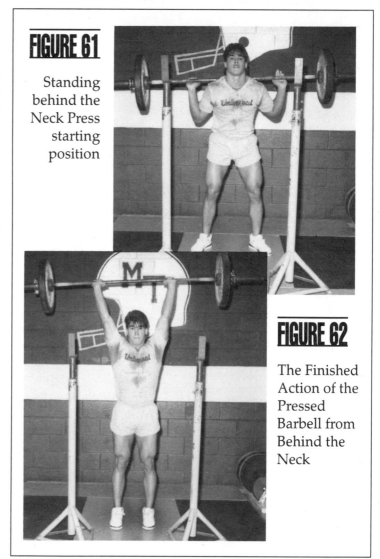

FIGURE 61 Standing behind the Neck Press starting position

FIGURE 62 The Finished Action of the Pressed Barbell from Behind the Neck

FRONT PRESS OR MILITARY PRESS (SEATED) - EXERCISE 6

STARTING POSITION

In the seated position, the barbell rests upon the top of the chest and shoulders with the grip in the desired position (Figure 63).

THE ACTION OF THE LIFT

As in the behind-the-neck press exercise, the same movement is repeated in this exercise with the barbell pressed in dynamic movement from the chest at a point above the head and then lowered back down into the starting position (Figure 64).

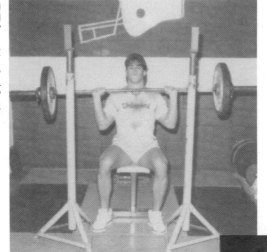

FIGURE 63

Seated Front Press starting position

SPEED-STRENGTH COACHING TIPS

Have the athletes check the bench they will be using. Remind the players that the trunk should remain still and that the bar's path travels in a vertical pattern.

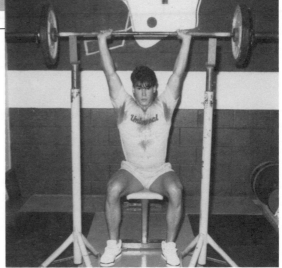

FIGURE 64

Barbell Pressed from chest to Arms Extension

PUSH PRESS (OR PUSH JERK) - EXERCISE 7

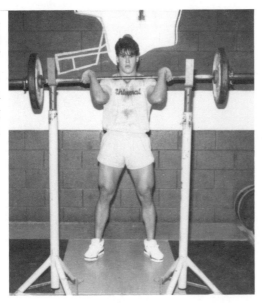

FIGURE 65

Push Press or Push Jerk starting position

STARTING POSITION

Take a medium or instructed grip position. Stand erect with the bar (at the shoulders-chest position) (Figure 65).

THE ACTION OF THE LIFT

Dip the knees about six inches and drive upward with the legs as the weight is pressed overhead. As the weight is moving up, drop under the bar to catch it overhead. Stand erect before the bar is lowered. The sequence of the action is dip-drive-dip. Lock the weight overhead and stand erect (Figures 66 and 67).

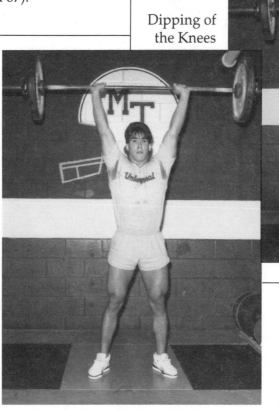

FIGURE 66

Dipping of the Knees

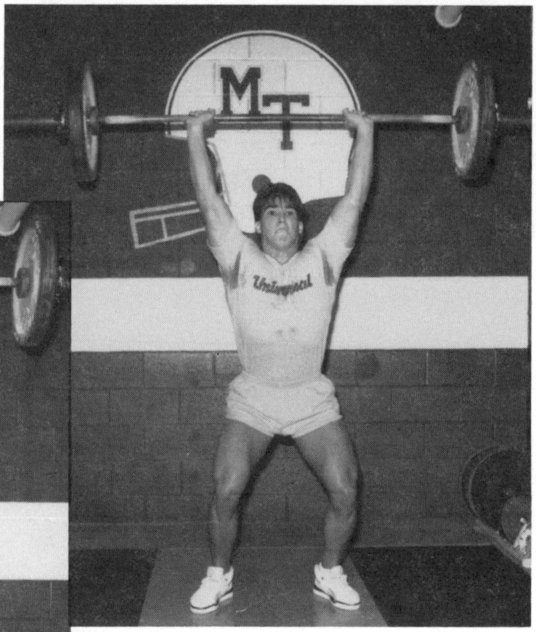

FIGURE 67

Standing erect in the Push or Push Jerk

SPEED STRENGTH COACHING TIPS

This is a good exercise for athletes who may be injured or due to some other circumstance cannot do the split jerk. Remind the athlete to hold for a two second count once the weight is positioned overhead.

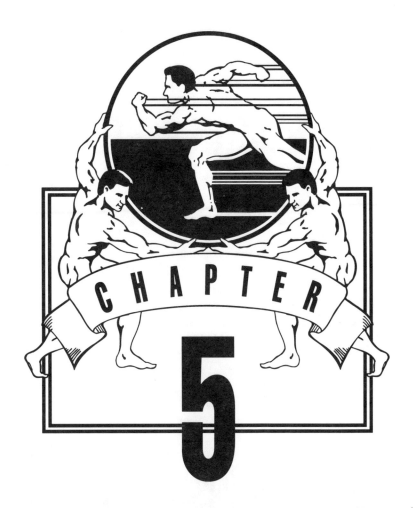

SQUATS AND LOWER BACK EXERCISES

"You can't ever work too much because there's no such thing as being in too good condition. You can't ever lift too many weights because you can't ever get too strong."
Dan Gable
Wrestler - Olympic Gold Medalist
College Wrestling Coach

SQUATS AND LOWER BACK EXERCISES

The squatting exercises have been called the foundation builder of athletic success. Without strong legs and hips, speed and strength development is minimal. As the squat strength increases, so does the speed-strength in other lifts. The squat thrives on hard work and gut-busting effort. This is why few conditioning programs succeed in this particular lift. There is no doubt that the bench press is far more enjoyable, but the results from squatting are what athletes' future may depend on. Coach Alvin Roy felt that if squatting exercises were incorporated into a proper program for running in the early high school years, the athlete's speed would increase as his strength from squats increased. Coach Roy used to say, *"The stronger I get, the faster I get."* The squat is definitely one of the foundation movements of speed-strength training for football players. It has elements of all four components included in the speed-strength concept.

BACK SQUAT-EXERCISE 1

STARTING POSITION

The feet are a little more than shoulder-width apart, with the toes turned slightly outward. The barbell is resting across the trapezius and back of the shoulders with arms in a comfortable position for balance. The grip may vary for balance (Figures 68A and 68B).

THE ACTION OF THE LIFT

Keep the head in a slightly raised, parallel position, with the eyes focusing slightly up, the back tight and the shoulders back. With the barbell centered over the hips, begin the squat down until the tops of the thighs are as low as is illustrated in Figure 69. From this low position, explode in a driving force upwards, returning to the

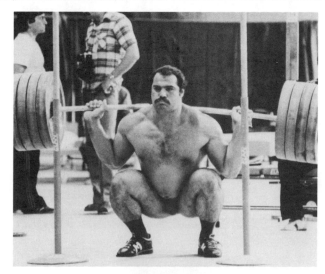

FIGURE 69

Top of the Thighs below parallel

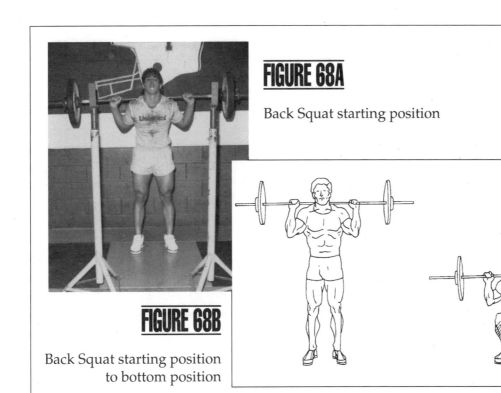

FIGURE 68A

Back Squat starting position

FIGURE 68B

Back Squat starting position to bottom position

starting position. Keep the chest up and the back tight through the entire movement. If the athletes are observed leaning forward as they come out of the bottom position, have them force the hips more under the bar while maintaining the head up and chest expanded.

SPEED-STRENGTH COACHING TIPS

The back in the squat is kept flat, but not vertical. The back squat develops the hips and leg power, as well as back strength, knee ligament strength, and aids in the overall development of running speed, power and strength.

FRONT SQUAT-EXERCISE 2

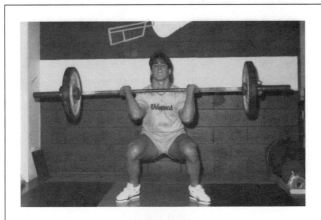

FIGURE 71

Front Squat with top of thighs below parallel

STARTING POSITION

The barbell should be resting across the front of the shoulders and on top of the chest. The feet are a little more than shoulder-width apart, with the toes turned outward slightly. The trunk is upright, and the barbell can be held in position with the grip in a comfortable position of balance with the elbows held high (Figures 70A and 70B).

THE ACTION OF THE LIFT

Keep the back as straight as possible. With the head up and back tight, squat down until the tops of the thighs are as low as illustrated in Figure 71. From this low position, explode in a

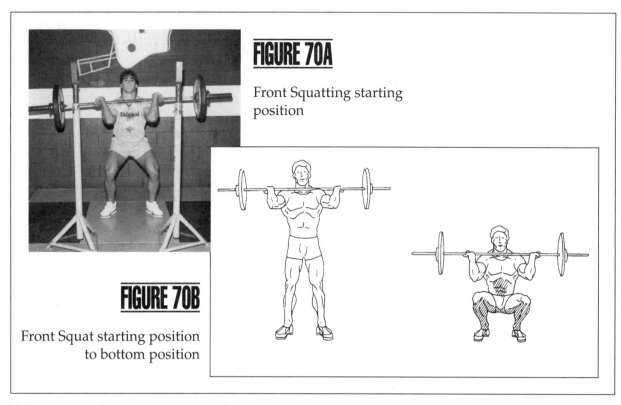

FIGURE 70A

Front Squatting starting position

FIGURE 70B

Front Squat starting position to bottom position

driving upward force, returning to the starting position. Keep the elbows up, shoulders square and the back tight throughout the entire front squat movement.

SPEED-STRENGTH COACHING TIPS

Review the coaching tips for the back squat. In the front squat, the weight is more in the front thigh area rather than the hips and is tremendously important in increasing hip flexibility if performed with proper form and technique. For athletes who cannot keep their heels on the floor in either the front or back squat, use a shaved wooden board or a five to ten pound plate under each heel. Remember to encourage athletes to hold their elbows high.

SPLIT SQUAT-EXERCISE 3

STARTING POSITION

This position, as illustrated in Figures 72A and 72B, is with the weight on the shoulders as in a back squat. Stride forward with one leg until the foot is in a good split position. The grip may vary for balance with each athlete.

THE ACTION OF THE LIFT

Start the movement down in a controlled lifting style until a deep split is reached, with the front knee ahead of the ankle and the front hip lower than the front knee and the rear leg nearly fully extended (Figure 73). Note that the trunk remains upright. Having recovered from the position by tilting the barbell slightly backwards and pushing off the rear leg as a prop, push vigorously with the front leg. Count the repetitions on the left leg and right leg together for a set.

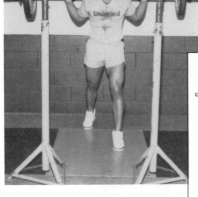

FIGURE 72A

Split Squat starting position

FIGURE 72B

Split Squat starting position to extension

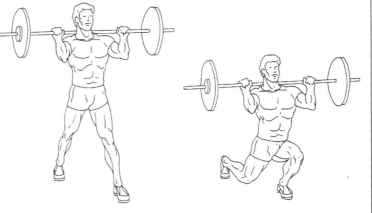

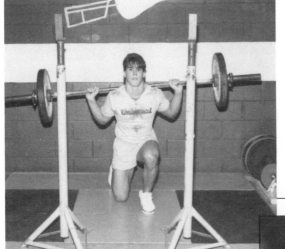

FIGURE 73

Action of the Split Squat Extension

SPEED-STRENGTH COACHING TIPS

Before starting, make certain the athletes are well balanced in the starting position. All sports which use lunging movements followed by very rapid and dynamic recovery will benefit from the employment of this exercise. This exercise can also be incorporated with dumbbells held in each hand and repeated in the same form and method. This super movement improves flexibility of the hips and the ankles.

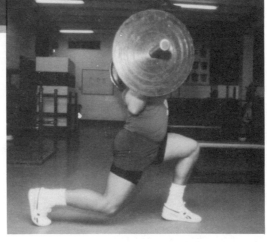

Split Squat Extension side view

ONE-LEGGED SQUAT-EXERCISE 4

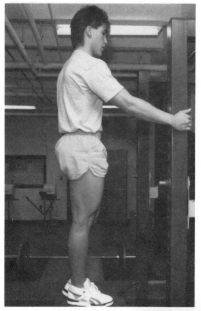

FIGURE 74

One-legged Squat starting position

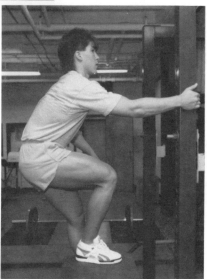

FIGURE 75

Downward movement of the One-legged Squat

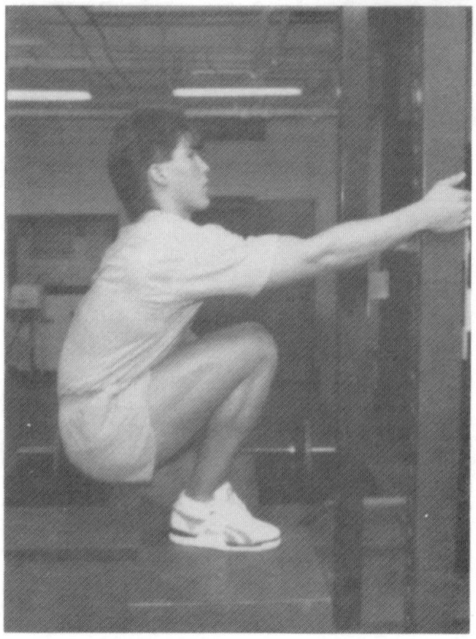

STARTING POSITION

Standing on top of the platform assume the position illustrated in Figure 74. Holding onto the side of the rack or stand with one leg hanging off and one leg in the squat support position, start downward in the back squat style.

THE ACTION OF THE LIFT

The body is lowered down, while holding onto the rack, as illustrated in Figure 75. By bending the support leg in the squat style, the body is lowered to a point where the calf muscle and hamstring are touching each other (Figure 76). Upon making the finishing movement, explode upward, back to the starting position.

SPEED-STRENGTH COACHING TIPS

This is an excellent warm-up exercise. Not only is the flexibility increased but also the full-range of movement. This exercise can be used with dumbbells and as an in-season competitive period exercise. It can also be modified and used as an excellent knee injury rehabilitation exercise.

FIGURE 76

Finishing position in the One-legged Squat

LUNGE-EXERCISE 5

STARTING POSITION

The starting position is the same as in the back squat. The athlete strides forward with one leg until the foot is in a good split position. The grip may vary for balance with each athlete.

THE ACTION OF THE LIFT

The action is the same as in the split squat exercise. The difference between the two exercises is that each repetition in the lunge is alternated from one leg to the other. For counting repetitions, one would be left leg than back to the starting position and then right leg and back to the starting position and so on (see Figure A).

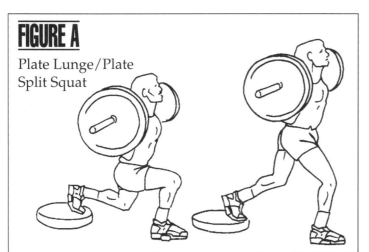

FIGURE A
Plate Lunge/Plate Split Squat

SPEED-STRENGTH COACHING TIPS

This exercise is really good for athletes who need to improve their balance, athletic coordination and foot work. The use of the plate may help in great strength and leg development by having the back leg up just a little higher. The force is then greater on the lead leg (see Figure A).

STEP-UPS / DUMBBELLS -- EXERCISE 6

STARTING POSITION

The dumbbells are gripped in each hand. The athlete faces the platforms to be used in the step-up exercise with the weight equally distributed throughout the body (see Figure B).

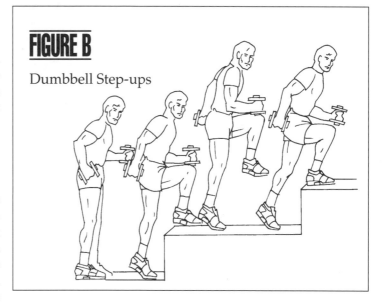

FIGURE B
Dumbbell Step-ups

THE ACTION OF THE LIFT

As illustrated in the figure, the athlete must drive the knee up and be able to place the foot to the surface of the first platform. As the contact is made with the foot to the platform, the athlete drives the other leg and knee into a ninety degree angle to the waist. This is very similar to the Running A's movement, except the athlete steps up and down and uses dumbbells.

After the opposite leg has moved to the waist, the athlete must bring his leg back down to the new height. Then repeat the movement again with the same leg for the desired number of repetitions to be used (see Figure B).

SPEED-STRENGTH COACHING TIPS

This movement works really well with more than one step. For years the one step has been used, but the three step approach gives the athlete greater follow through and quicker reaction strength development because of the repetition and not having to go back to the floor and start the exercise over again. Again, this is an excellent movement for balance, coordination and body control. Also for players who do not have the developed leg drives, this is a super addition to the back and front squat exercises. As pictured in the figure, the three step platform of steps works better and develops greater speed-strength because of the operated movement from step to step (see Figure B).

STEP-UPS/BARBELL - EXERCISE 7

STARTING POSITION

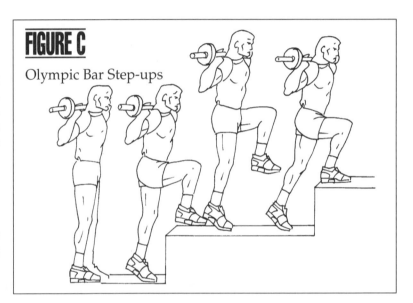

FIGURE C
Olympic Bar Step-ups

The barbell is fixed in the starting position as used in the back squat, split squat and the lunge exercises. Again, the athlete is facing the platform to be used in the step-up exercise (see Figure C).

THE ACTION OF THE LIFT

This exercise is the same as the step-up dumbbell drill in its basic action (see Figure C).

SPEED-STRENGTH COACHING TIPS

Remind the athlete to keep the torso upright and shoulders back. Balance is a real key to perfecting this exercise. Again, the three step approach will give the athlete faster results in developing leg and knee drive for running and jumping. This is a super assistance exercise with other squatting exercises.

HYPEREXTENSION EXERCISE

The hyperextension exercise is an excellent lower back and lower torso strengthener. Strengthening of the lower torso increases flexibility and improves a player's body control (lowering and raising) and develops muscles for protection of the back from possible injury.

EXERCISE 1

STARTING POSITION

Assume the position in Figure 77 of lying flat with the stomach over the hyperextension bench or with the feet held securely, or (as seen in Figure 78) against a wall and the hips supported solidly so the upper body can hang over the support. Lock the arms around the back of the head.

THE ACTION OF THE LIFT

From the hanging position in Figure 77, lift the head and extend the upper body so the shoulders and head come as high above the hips as possible and hold for a two-second count at parallel; then lower back to the hang position. Lifting the chest as high as possible makes sure the athlete gets a solid contraction from the lower back muscles.

SPEED-STRENGTH COACHING TIPS

As in Figure 79, the athlete is holding the weight resistance behind at the back of the neck or head. Start with this exercise using no weight resistance, but as the player becomes more accustomed to the exercise, resistance should be added. Different weighted medicine balls are excellent to use.

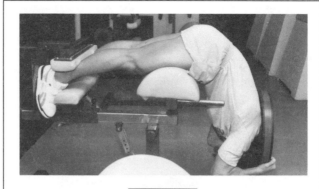

FIGURE 77

Hyperextension starting position with Weight Resistance

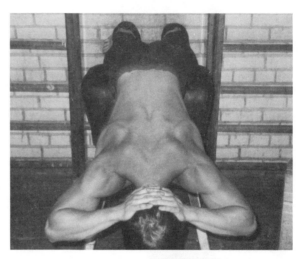

FIGURE 78

A makeshift Hyperextension

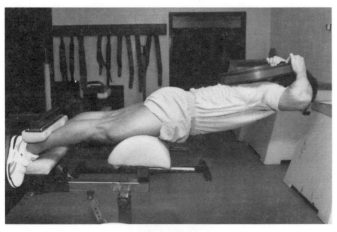

FIGURE 79

The use of weight for additional resistance

GLUTE HAM RAISE EXERCISE

The glute ham raise exercise develops the muscles in the following: (1) lower back, (2) gluteus maximums and (3) hamstrings all in one exercise. This is an excellent exercise to develop the speed muscles of the legs and the speed-strength necessary to improve the starting and reaction strength of each player. It is one of the best exercises for working the muscles of a football player's buttocks, hamstring and lower back.

EXERCISE 1

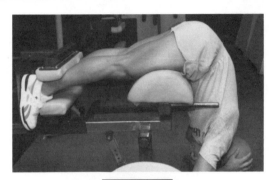

FIGURE 80

Glute Ham Raise starting position

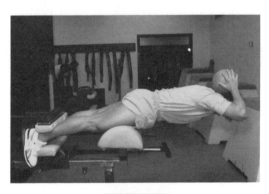

FIGURE 81

Action movement of the Glute Ham Raise

STARTING POSITION

Repeat the position used in the hyperextension. The incorporation of the glute ham chair has advanced the glute ham raise (Figure 80)

THE ACTION OF THE LIFT

As illustrated in Figure 81, the movement is identical to the hyperextension exercise, except in the hyperextension the athlete stops at parallel. In the glute ham raise, he keeps going until the hamstring and legs are in a ninety-degree position (Figure 82). This action incorporates the hamstring muscles into a maximum muscle contraction of a speed-strength movement.

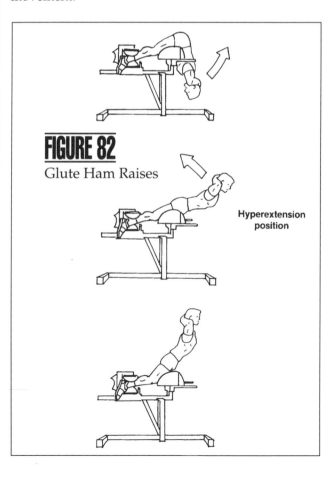

FIGURE 82

Glute Ham Raises

SPEED-STRENGTH COACHING TIPS

As illustrated in Figure 82, the movement from parallel to ninety degrees will help in the hamstring development. This exercise is often overlooked in speed-strength devel-opment programs.

See additional exercises that are different yet use the glute ham movement (Figure A and B).

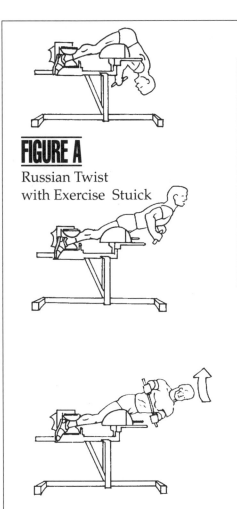

FIGURE A
Russian Twist with Exercise Stuick

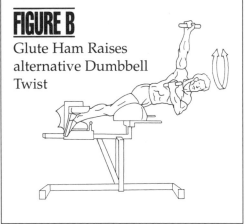

FIGURE B
Glute Ham Raises alternative Dumbbell Twist

GOOD MORNING EXERCISES

The good morning exercise is a fine back strengthener and has three variations. The exercise is a full-range movement and will be a very important remedial exercise. In the beginning, it is wise to move smoothly and under control in both the flexing and extending movements, but as strength is developed, the extension part of the movement should become more dynamic.

GOOD MORNING (STANDING) EXERCISE 1

STARTING POSITION

Repeat the standing squat position, feet a little over medium-width apart and the barbell resting on the shoulders behind the neck. Use the same position as in the back squat exercise. The medium grip position is the best for controlling and balancing the bar (Figure 83).

THE ACTION OF THE LIFT

From the upright athletic standing position, squat about a quarter of the way down, then curl forward so that the spine is rounded. The legs are not really in a locked-out position, but are slightly bent to relieve tension on the hamstring muscles. From this parallel position, uncurl the body back to the starting position. Keep the back tight and the neck "bulled" against the bar (Figure 84 A and B).

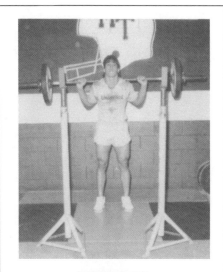

FIGURE 83

Standing Good Morning starting position

67

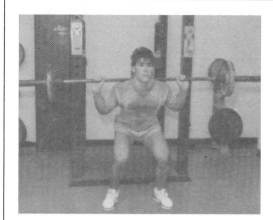

FIGURE 84A

Quarter Squat Position

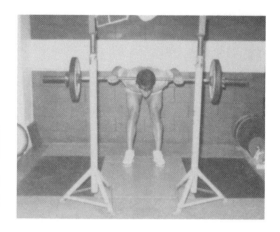

FIGURE 84B

Action of the lift in the Standing Good Morning

SPEED-STRENGTH COACHING TIPS

The importance of lower back strength will show far greater development and improvement in the football player. The great strength of the lower back enables the young athlete to build as protection fine, hard muscles in a very vulnerable area of the human body. Both small and large muscles surrounding the spine are strengthened by the good morning exercise.

GOOD MORNING (SEATED/BENT LEGS OR STRAIGHT)-EXERCISE 2

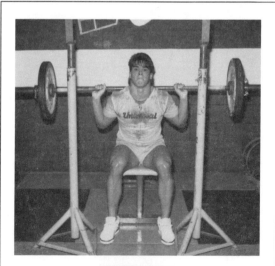

FIGURE 85

Seated Good Morning bent legs starting position

STARTING POSITION

In the seated position, the barbell rests upon the shoulders behind the neck. The grip is a little wider than medium-width, but it may also be widened farther for better coordination and balance (Figure 85 and 86).

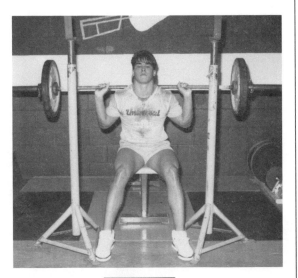

FIGURE 86

Seated Good Morning straight legs starting position

THE ACTION OF THE LIFT

The action of the lift is no different from that of the standing good morning exercise. This is a more controllable movement and is excellent for athletes in rehabilitation (Figures 87 and 88).

SPEED-STRENGTH COACHING TIPS

This is a key movement that teaches the athlete how to flex and extend the lower back, which plays such an important part in the development of football ability.

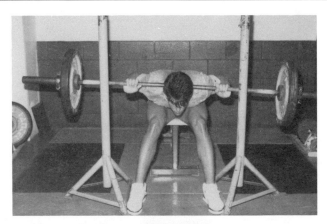

FIGURE 87

Bent legs action of the Lift

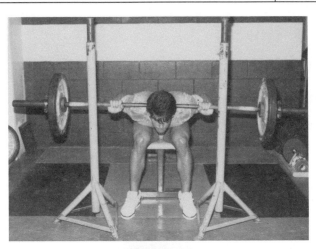

FIGURE 88

Straight legs action of the Lift

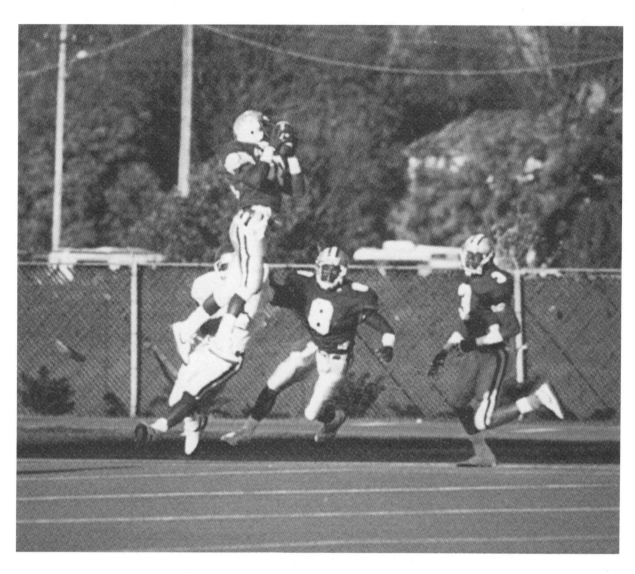

"Psych for the maximum"
E. J. "Doc" Kreis

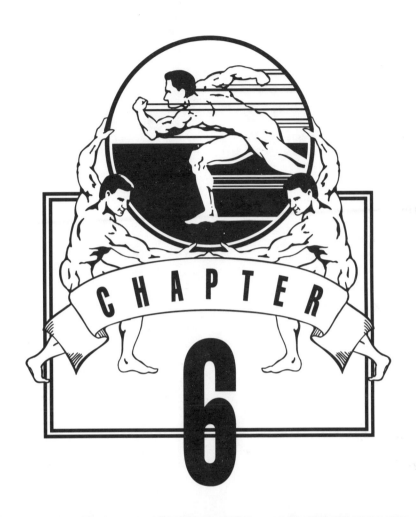

CHAPTER 6

THE EXTRA EXERCISE ESSENTIALS: GYMNASTIC MOVEMENT AND ABDOMINAL/NECK EXERCISE

"It's very hard to predict where the limits are."
Grete Waitz
Distance Running

THE EXTRA EXERCISE ESSENTIALS: GYMNASTIC MOVEMENT AND ABDOMINAL/NECK EXERCISE

Gymnastics was the birth place of weight resistance exercises, and these exercises are still valuable to trainer or coach in the development of his football players. The importance of the gymnastic exercises is that they teach the athlete to control his body. These simple, but difficult, exercises have been the base for athletic progress. It is the belief of this writer that programs of speed-strength training must teach and train athletes to master their body's weight. The only way to be able to achieve these movements is to practice. They are definite strength builders.

CHIN-UP-EXERCISE 1

STARTING POSITION

Assume a hanging position on the chin-up bar, palms forward using a medium grip. Then allow the body to drop into a hanging position (Figure 89).

THE ACTION OF THE LIFT

Make a good even pull with the shoulders and arms, bringing the chest up to the bar before lowering the body back to the starting position. Try to keep the body as naturally loose and straight as possible (Figure 90).

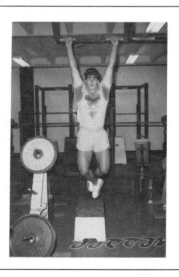

FIGURE 89

Chin-up starting position

SPEED-STRENGTH COACHING TIPS

Many variations of chinning exercises may be used by varying the different grip positions. Increasing the resistance of both the pull and return to starting positions offers other variations.

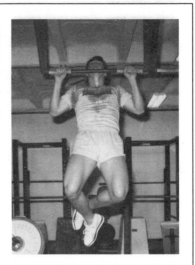

FIGURE 90

Chin to Bar then to chest

PARALLEL BAR DIPS - EXERCISE 2

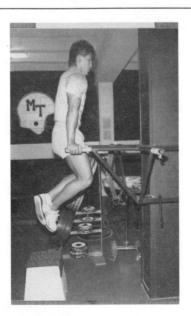

FIGURE 91

Parallel Bar Dips starting position

STARTING POSITION

Assume the starting portion between the bars as shown in Figure 91.

THE ACTION OF THE LIFT

Lower the body by bending the arms and chest down until the elbows in relation to the shoulders are almost in a ninety-degree angle (Figure 92). Upon completion, return to the starting position by pressing with the arm and shoulder muscles back and up to arms' length.

SPEED-STRENGTH COACHING TIPS

The upright position of the athlete while executing the dips places more stress on the triceps. When the athlete leans forward, there will be more movement of the deltoids and pectorals. As in the case of any gymnastic strength movement, greater resistance can be added by using dumbbells and weight plates.

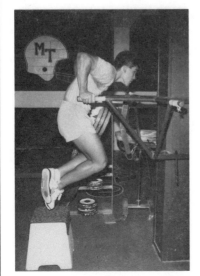

FIGURE 92

Elbows almost in a 90-Degree angle

BALLISTIC PUSH-UP—EXERCISE 3

STARTING POSITION

Assume the position, as illustrated in Figure 93, with arms and feet planted on top of the platform.

THE ACTION OF THE LIFT

Lower the body by bending the arms and dropping down between the two platforms (Figure 94).

To start the push-up, repeat the downward push and explode upward by pushing off the floor with the arms and shoulders.

SPEED-STRENGTH COACHING TIPS

This exercise begins as a regular push-up drill. After the regular push-ups are completed, start the football player with two-by-four platforms and work up to heights of eighteen inches maximum.

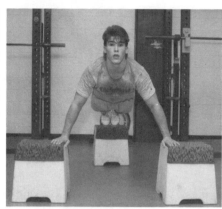

FIGURE 93
Ballistic Push-up starting position

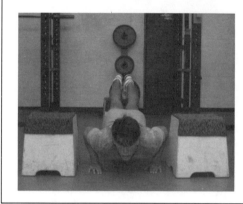

FIGURE 94
the Drop Between the Boxes

ABDOMINAL AND NECK EXERCISES

The abdominal muscle region is the most highly visible area of the athletic body, yet may be the most overlooked and underworked region in strength development programs for athletes.

Using speed-strength on the waist and abdominal areas coordinates all parts of the body. The waist and abdominal area contain about one-third of the body weight. Failure to develop strength and flexibility in the rotational muscles of the lower back is one of the major causes of low back strains and pains among athletes in football.

The development of abdominal strength is important to the athlete. The abdominal region is only as strong as the weakest link. The exercises listed and described are some of the best that can be incorporated into a speed-strength program.

SIT-UP WITH RESISTANCE AND SIT-UP WITHOUT RESISTANCE--EXERCISE I

STARTING POSITION

Assume the supine position on the floor. If someone cannot hold the feet down, then look for a bench or barbell to serve the same function. When used, the weight resistance is placed behind the head. Weight plates, dumbbells and medicine balls are excellent resistance implements (Figure 95).

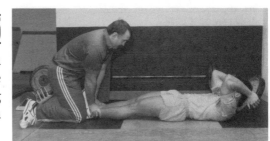

FIGURE 95 Sit-up with Resistance starting position

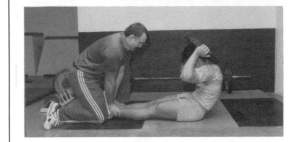

FIGURE 96 The action of the lift as the athlete moves forward and up using the abdominal muscles

THE ACTION OF THE LIFT

Sit up by reaching forward with the head and attempt to touch the knees with the forehead. Try to keep the legs as straight as possible.

The knees will bend a little as the athlete drives forward and upward. Keep the abdominals tight going up and down (Figure 96).

SPEED-STRENGTH COACHING TIPS

Use some form of weight resistance after the initial sit-up has been mastered. This exercise is excellent for the development of the abdominal muscles, including hip and spinal flexion.

SIT-UP HYPEREXTENDED—EXERCISE 2

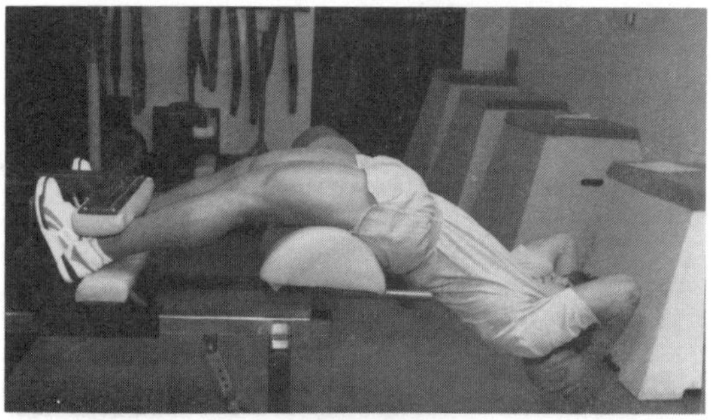

STARTING POSITION

Assume the starting position, as illustrated in Figure 97, extending the body backward while maintaining the hips in a fixed position. Notice that hyperextension is achieved in the Glute Ham Chair. This exercise can be performed over any apparatus where the feet and hips can be fixed (Figure 98).

THE ACTION OF THE LIFT

From the hyperextended position, sit up to a point of full flexion. Then return under control to the starting position (Figure 99).

SPEED-STRENGTH COACHING TIPS

This is a more advanced abdominal exercise. The use of weight resistance is not for the beginning football player. Since this is an advanced abdominal exercise, other movements of a simpler nature should be completed before using this exercise in training.

FIGURE 97

Sit-up Hyperextension starting position

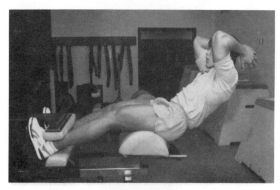

FIGURE 98

Upward movement of the Hyperextesion Sit-up

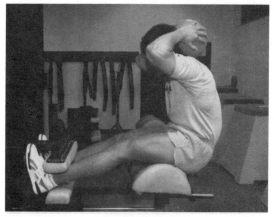

FIGURE 99

Finish position of the Hyperextension Sit-up

HANGING BENT KNEE/STRAIGHT LEGS RAISE--EXERCISE 3

STARTING POSITION

Repeat the hanging position using the chin-up medium grip (Figure 100).

THE ACTION OF THE LIFT

Begin by letting the body hang straight down from the bar. Pull the knees to the chest and then try to curl the hips by pulling the knees high and rounding the back. Lift the legs up parallel and hold for a two-second count. Lower the legs under control to keep from rocking until the body is hanging before repeating the exercise (Figures 101).

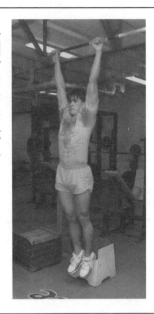

FIGURE 100
Hanging Bent Knee/Straight Legs Raise starting position

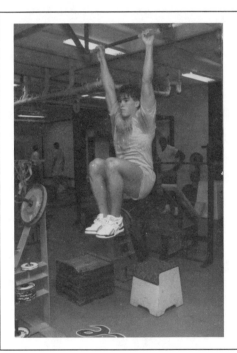

FIGURE 101
Bent Knee

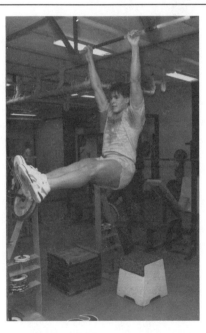

FIGURE 102
Straight Leg Raise from the starting position

SPEED-STRENGTH COACHING TIPS

The straight-legged raises from this position may be used to develop the hip flexions which are necessary for high knee action in running. It helps to have someone support the lower back while working this exercise.

DUMBBELL SIDE BEND—EXERCISE 4

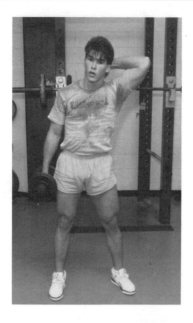

FIGURE 103
Starting position of Dumbbell Side Bend

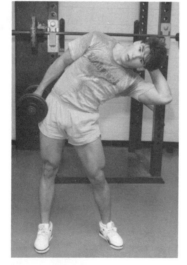

FIGURE 104
The action of the Side Bend

FIGURE 105
The Action of the Side Bend

STARTING POSITION

Hold the dumbbell in one hand; place the feet about one foot farther apart than hip-width and keep the knees braced as illustrated in Figure 103.

THE ACTION OF THE LIFT

The body is bent strongly over to the opposite side by lateral flexion of the trunk. With the hips positioned slightly forward, lean laterally to the side of the dumbbell. The opposite hand is placed behind the head (Figure 104).

SPEED-STRENGTH COACHING TIPS

Try to perform this exercise while maintaining the proper stance. Setting the hips slightly forward in the starting position prevents the athlete from bending forward. Remember to keep the feet flat and knees braced. Make sure that the exercise involves both sides of the trunk.

NOTE:

The following illustrations are additional special Exercises for the abdominal muscles

GLUTE CHAIR RAISES
WITH MEDICINE BALL-SIT-UPS

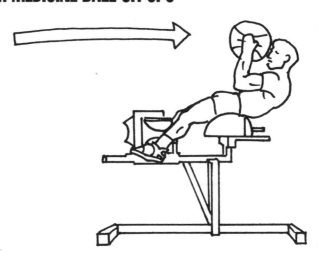

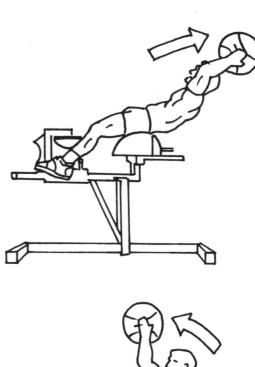

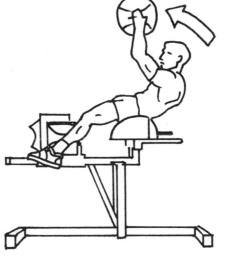

SEATED, BEHIND NECK WEIGHT TWIST

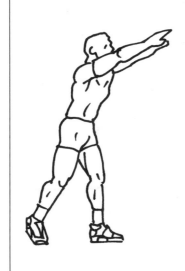

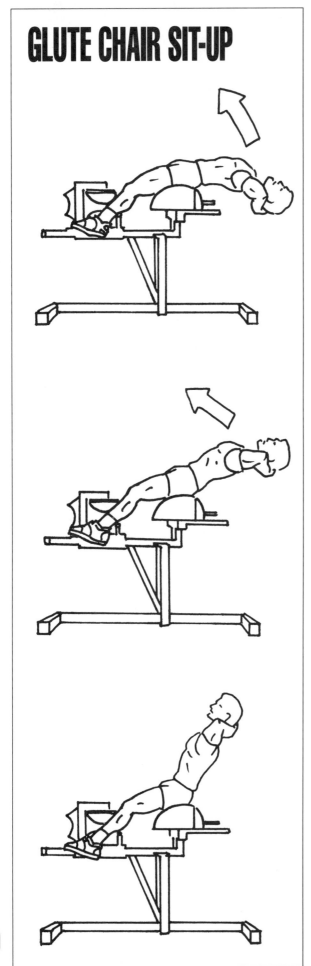
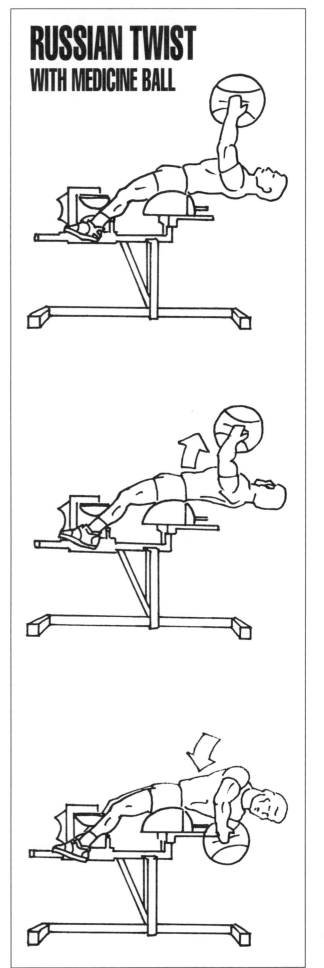

NECK EXERCISES

The neck has already been exercised a number of times by the previous exercises. The snatches, cleans and pressing movements are dynamic builders of the neck area. The better developed the trapezius muscles become, the more the protection for the athlete. Following are additional special exercises for the neck.

WRESTLER'S BRIDGE-EXERCISE 1

STARTING POSITION

This exercise can be performed while on the front or on the back. Lying on the back, slowly arch upwards (Figure 106), keeping the weight on the heels and the back of the head.

THE ACTION OF THE LIFT

Place the body's weight on the heels and the back of the head. This helps the athlete generate the amount of weight and pressure the neck can absorb. Rock under control back

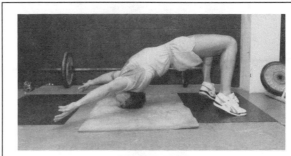

FIGURE 106

Wrestler's Bridge starting position on the Back

and forth so that the nose touches the floor. Then straighten the body out again. The front bridge is performed in similar form, except that the pressure is on the forehead and toes. The use of hands against thighs helps balance and support (Figure 107).

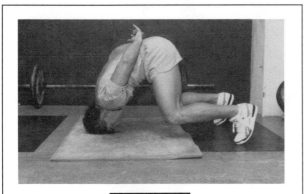

FIGURE 107

The Front Bridge

SPEED-STRENGTH COACHING TIPS

Both versions of the wrestler's bridge are tough exercises and should not be completed without some form of slow warm-up at the beginning.

NECK HARNESS-EXERCISE 2

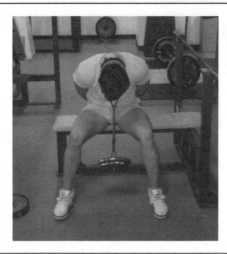

FIGURE 108
Neck Harness starting position

STARTING POSITION

The neck harness apparatus is placed over the head and is hanging down over the head. Once the weight implements are loaded, the neck is free to support the weight in a freehanging position with the neck slightly extended forward (Figure 108).

THE ACTION OF THE LIFT

The action of the neck movement is usually completed by lowering and raising the neck. Again, the amount of weight is not as important as the range of motion (Figure 109).

SPEED-STRENGTH COACHING TIPS

The use of neck harness, helmets with weights attached to them and force resistance of manual pressure are all excellent little extras that help develop the muscles of the neck.

Remember that the incorporation of the snatch movements, cleans and presses have already started the neck strength development in the speed-strength training program.

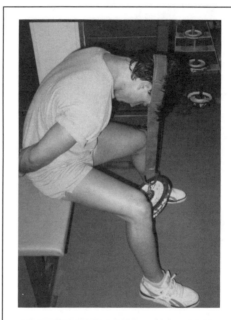

FIGURE 109
Lowering and then raising using the neck only

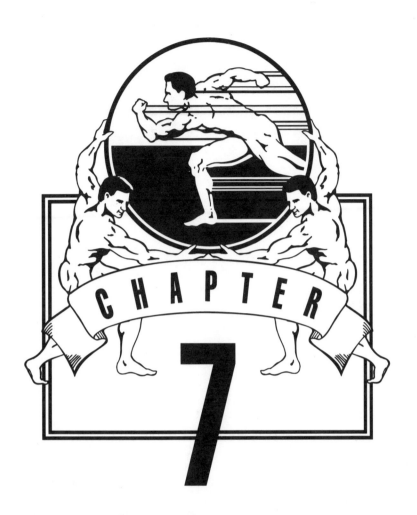

PLYOMETRICS-LOWER BODY EXPLOSIVENESS

"They can because they think they can."
Virgil
Greek Poet

PLYOMETRICS-LOWER BODY EXPLOSIVENESS

Plyometrics is a form of emphasis training that revolves around the jump movement. In the Soviet Union, there is no word like plyometrics; these jumps are simply called "hit" and "shock," while United States trainers call these same movements jump and depth jump. Plyometric jumping incorporates different forms such as: (1) jumps for height, (2) jumps for distance, (3) single leg jumps, (4) double leg jumps, (5) hops, (6) depth jumps with a single, double, or triple rebound effect, (7) reaction speed-strength plyometrics and (8) reaction speed-strength sprinting skills. Some actions are singular in nature, and some work in series, sets or combinations. Although acceptance of plyometrics has been relatively slow in the United States, the use of plyometrics is gradually finding its way into professional, college and high school conditioning programs. With speed-strength training emphasizing starting, reaction and explosive strength, the competitive edge is being gained by those who have utilized plyometrics as another way to vastly improve their athletes.

Plyometric movements help improve the quickness and explosiveness of the athlete. When an athlete improves his vertical, horizontal and reaction strength, his starting and explosive strength also improve. Thus, the level of absolute strength is improved for the football athlete.

LOWER BODY EXPLOSIVENESS

Today, speed is even more a measure of successful competition. To develop lower body explosive strength, an excellent leg speed-strength program should complement weight training. Jumping, depth jumps, hopping, bounding and squat jumps contribute to explosive leg strength. This approach helps develop faster movement in starting, reaction speed and greater speed-strength. The coach or trainer can review in this chapter different exercises involving plyometric movements and select from ten different drills used for the development of speed-strength. Coaches should be sure when planning speed-strength training during main competitive period to allow two days off from heavy plyometrics exercises before a game.

JUMPING DRILLS

Incorporating jumps into a training program is the simplest form of plyometrics. Jumping involves either one leg or both legs or even alternating between legs. It is better to start off beginning football players with double leg jumps until the legs are accustomed to the jumping movements. It is important that the trainer/coach remember that the amount of force generated in a single leg jump is about twice that of double leg movement. If the young athlete's muscles are not prepared for this force, it could be injurious.

Jumping exercises can be used to duplicate different heights and directions, as well as jumping onto and off various platforms. Jumping over an object becomes more effective for the football player than simple jumping because it forces the athlete to jump a little higher which, in turn, creates greater force upon the landing. Jumping over different heights and obstacles allows for a progressive development that in time will allow the athlete to jump even higher. The nervous system is exposed to different amounts of force from different jumps, which provides for greater leg explosiveness and development. The following ten plyometric drills serve as examples of the types of jumps that the coach/trainer may use in his speed-strength training program.

DRILL 1: PLATFORM JUMP

STARTING POSITION

Assume a solid standing position with the pressure on the balls of the feet and knees slightly bent. Using the arms as balancing factors, prepare the mind "psyche" for maximum explosion upwards and onto the platform (Figure 110).

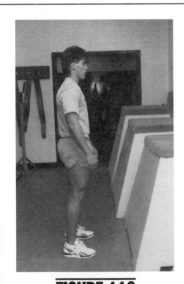

FIGURE 110

Platform Jump starting position

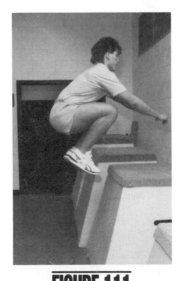

FIGURE 111

Jump movement upward

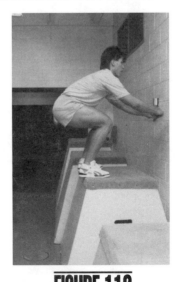

FIGURE 112

Landing form the Jump Off Floor

THE ACTION OF THE MOVEMENT

From the explosion upward and forward slightly, the amount of force will allow the athlete to land on both feet on top of the jumping platform. Upon landing, the athlete may repeat the platform jump exercise or the depth jump followed by platform jumping to another platform (Figure 111 and 112).

SPEED-STRENGTH COACHING TIPS

This is an outstanding exercise for beginning athletes who have a strength weakness in the lower body. The starting height should be eighteen to thirty-six inches, depending on the level of the athlete.

I recommend the following workout program for a football player: (1) three sets of six repetitions; (2) one time a week during the competitive period (in-season); and (3) two to three times a week during the preparatory phase (off-season).

DRILL 2: OVER THE TOP SIDE JUMP

STARTING POSITION

Standing erect, place the feet a heel's distance apart (Figure 110), with the knees slightly bent.

THE ACTION OF THE MOVEMENT

Stand to the side of the blocking bag (approximately twelve to eighteen inches high) and hop back and forth over the blocking bag, landing on both feet each time (Figure 113).

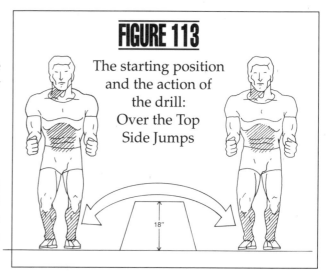

FIGURE 113

The starting position and the action of the drill: Over the Top Side Jumps

SPEED-STRENGTH COACHING TIPS

Quickness is important here, so keep a record of how many jumps are achieved in a recommended time period.

DRILL 3: STRADDLE BENCH JUMP

STARTING POSITION

Stand erect with the knees slightly bent, similar to the front or back squat starting position. The only difference is that the flat bench is being straddled (Figure 114).

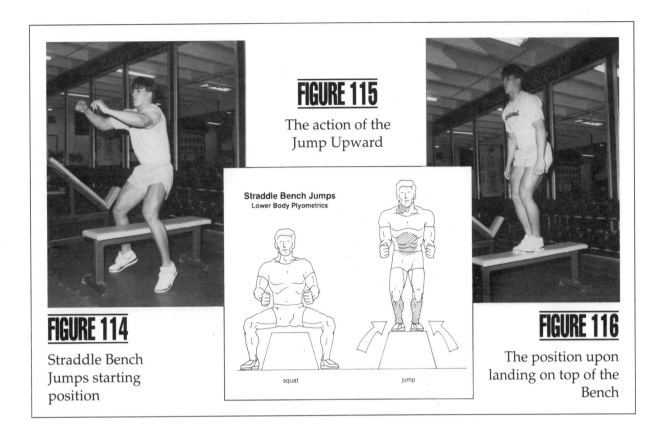

FIGURE 115 The action of the Jump Upward

FIGURE 114 Straddle Bench Jumps starting position

FIGURE 116 The position upon landing on top of the Bench

THE ACTION OF THE MOVEMENT

Use the double knee bend going downward until contact is made with the top of the bench. When contact is made, explode as quickly as possible in order to be able to have both feet land on top of the bench with full extension achieved; then return back down into the starting position. Repeat the process until the desired number of repetitions is completed (Figures 115 and 116).

SPEED-STRENGTH COACHING TIPS

This exercise can be performed with or without use of weight resistance. Remind the athletes to explode and try to land under control.

DEPTH JUMP DRILLS

Dr. Fred Hatfield and Dr. Michael Yessis feel that the most effective height for the depth jump is between thirty and forty inches. For beginning athletes, the coach should lower the height until the proper form and technique are mastered. Yessis and Hatfield also state that "as a general rule-of-thumb, your depth jump height should be no more than a foot above your vertical jumping ability." Depth jumping from too great a height should be avoided. Many beginners and second-year players usually function on the principle that "the more I do, the better I get," and because of these ideas, they increase the height to amounts that are beyond their capabilities.

When you jump from too high a height, there is too much flexion in the legs, which absorb most of the force of the landing, and thus there is very little force to propel you upwards. You thus end up with a weaker lower jump. Jumping from too high a height also involves different take off mechanisms. It is also important to keep in mind that it is most advantageous to execute depth jumps after adequate strength preparation (preparatory period of training). Practice has shown that in most cases you should be able to squat 2.5 times your body weight before undertaking maximum depth jumps (Yessis & Hatfield).

DRILL 4: DEPTH JUMP

STARTING POSITION

Assume the starting position on top of the platform (Figure 117).

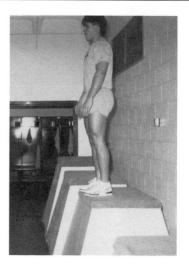

FIGURE 117

Depth Jump starting position

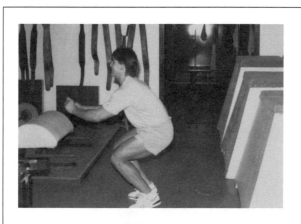

FIGURE 118

The landing on the Depth Jump

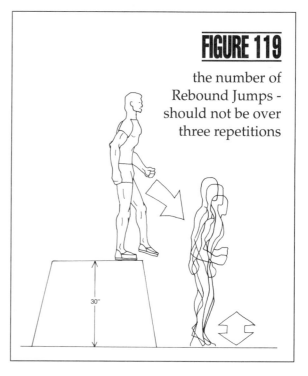

FIGURE 119

the number of Rebound Jumps - should not be over three repetitions

THE ACTION OF THE MOVEMENT

When stepping off the platform, the athlete will drop straight down, landing on both feet together at the same time. As he makes contact with the surface, the immediate action is to jump straight upward and slightly forward, obtaining as much height as possible on each jump.

Upon landing, try and be as vertical as possible so that the maximum load can be placed on the leg muscles. The landing should first be on the balls of both feet and then on the whole foot, followed by the ankle, knee and joint flexion (Figure 118).

SPEED-STRENGTH COACHING TIPS

Remember to use a good landing surface. The number of rebound jumps repeated should not be over three repetitions (Figure 119).

A recommended workout for a football player includes: (1) two sets of five repetitions with a triple rebound, (2) one time a week during main-competitive period (in-season) and (3) two-three times a week during the preparatory phase (off-season). The coach should allow two days off before a game.

DRILL 5: SHOCK JUMP

STARTING POSITION

As in depth jump, assume the starting position on top of the platform.

THE ACTION OF THE MOVEMENT

The movement is the same action used for the depth jump. As the football player steps off and makes contact with the surface, the action is completed. The landing should be in an upright position with feet wide apart and knees slightly bent in a ready position so that the maximum load can be placed on the leg muscles. The landing should first be on the balls of the feet, transferring the weight to each foot, followed by ankle, knee and hip joint flexion (Figure 120). The knees are in the bent athletic position with a wider base.

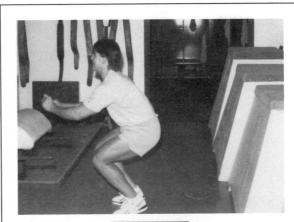

FIGURE 120
The Landing of a Shock Jump

SPEED-STRENGTH COACHING TIPS

1. Remember to use a proper landing surface.
2. Use the prime movers of the legs and hips to absorb the major force.
3. Flex on the landing.

HOPPING DRILLS

The hopping drills are excellent for developing overall coordination, balance, agility and arm position. Also, the amount of work force that is placed on each leg teaches the athlete's body awareness and control.

DRILL 6: FRONT HURDLE HOPS

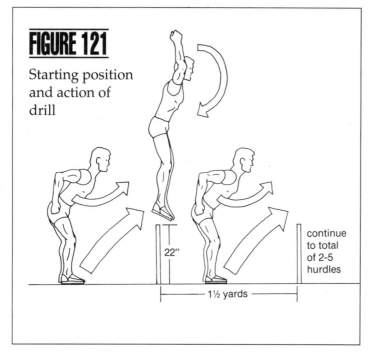

FIGURE 121
Starting position and action of drill

STARTING POSITION

Take a standing position on both feet in front of the first hurdle to be hopped (Figure 121).

ACTION OF THE MOVEMENT

Jump over the hurdle and land on both feet. Then quickly repeat the jump up and over the next four hurdles until the last hurdle is cleared (Figure 121). The arms should help the athlete balance and coordinate the movement. The arms are both driven upward as the hop occurs. The action is to maximize height, not distance.

SPEED-STRENGTH COACHING TIPS

The idea is to spend as little time as possible on the ground between hurdles. Athletes should not wear weighted vest or ankle weights in this drill. The drill consists of five hurdles spread one and one-half yards apart. Start with the hurdles at the lowest level and slowly move the hurdles up as the athlete makes improvements.

DRILL 7: DOUBLE LEG HOPS

STARTING POSITION

Assume the standing position used in front hurdle hops (Figure 122).

THE ACTION OF THE MOVEMENT

Similar to the standing long jump, the action is to maximize distance, not height. Upon landing, quickly repeat the hopping motion for the required distance (Figure 122).

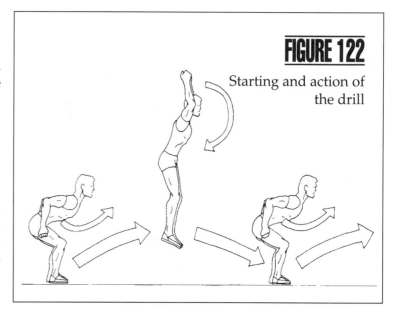

FIGURE 122
Starting and action of the drill

SPEED-STRENGTH COACHING TIPS

Again, the idea is to spend as little time as possible on the ground between double-leg hops. Require good form and technique. These hops are recommended for use in the warm-up plan. This is a very simple movement and is excellent for beginning athletes to use in warm-up drills before weight training, as well as for warm-down after finishing drills.

DRILL 8: SINGLE LEG HOP

STARTING POSITION

Stand erect in a relaxed position.

THE ACTION OF THE MOVEMENT

Thrust forward and upward with the right knee and at the same time hop forward on the left leg. The action is repeated several times for a given distance. The action of the left arm is held up in proper running form and uses a pumping movement back and forth. The right arm serves as a balance of control to help in the hopping action. The landing should be flat-footed on the ground (Figure 123).

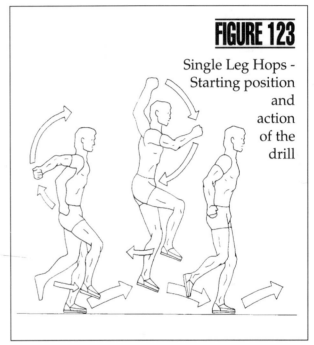

FIGURE 123

Single Leg Hops - Starting position and action of the drill

SPEED-STRENGTH COACHING TIPS

The arms should help the athlete balance and coordinate the movement. The difficult part is not only hopping on one leg, but keeping the other leg up as high as possible in readiness for the next hop. The single leg hops are an excellent exercise for leg coordination and speed quickness development of the football player.

SQUAT JUMP DRILL

Jumping exercises with weights are a different method that can be employed to increase the explosive speed-strength in football players. It is a good variation from the other forms of plyometrics exercise. The amount of weight should be no more than half of the athlete's body weight. It should allow for a smooth and controllable movements.

DRILL 9: SQUAT JUMP

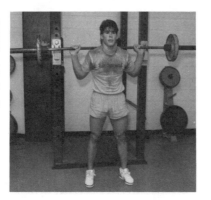

FIGURE 124
Starting Position in the Squat Jump

STARTING POSITION

Standing erect, the athlete positions himself with the barbell on his shoulders in the back squat position. Feet are shoulder width; the knees are slightly bent (Figure 124). Grip is slightly over medium.

THE ACTION OF THE MOVEMENT

Dipping slightly lower using the double knee bend, jump in an upward fashion off the surface. Make the force great enough to get full leg extension. Then prepare for a smooth, coordinated, balanced landing (Figures 125 and 126). Repeat the action for the given repetitions.

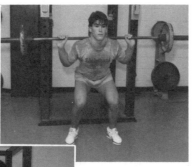

FIGURE 125
The Double Knee Bend Position

SPEED-STRENGTH COACHING TIPS

This exercise can be performed by using a dumbbell and can also be practiced using a barbell (Figure 127). This movement can be executed using either the squat or split squat procedure. Again use no more than half of the athlete's body weight as maximum poundage. This exercise is recommended for either or both periods of preparatory/competitive training.

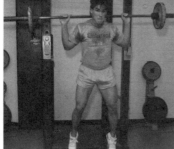

FIGURE 126
Jump and Extension

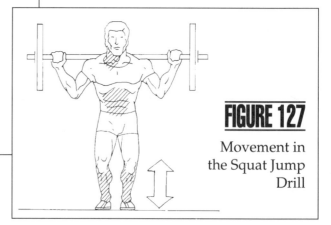

FIGURE 127
Movement in the Squat Jump Drill

REACTION SPEED-STRENGTH PLYOMETRIC DRILLS

This series of reaction speed-strength plyometric drills is designed to increase the reaction speed of the leap. *Track Coach Dean Hayes best explains reaction strength plyometric: *"These exercises help the legs learn to snap back off the ground more quickly, thus teaching you to automatically respond and increase faster improvement of reaction speed."* Over the years, Coach Hayes pioneered and formulated many concepts and ideas that have been implemented by world-class long and triple jumpers and sprinters alike. These drills have obvious benefits for football players and have become invaluable plyometric exercises.

These reaction strength plyometric drills are:(1) Hayes Double Leg Top Hop, (2) Hayes Double Leg in the Hole Hop, (3) Hayes Single Leg Top Hop and (4) Hayes Single Leg in the Hole Hop. These drills will make a difference in the improvement of speed development.

DRILL 1: HAYES DOUBLE LEG TOP HOPS

STARTING POSITION

As in the platform jumps, assume squat stance starting position.

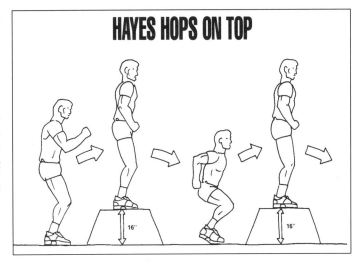

THE ACTION OF THE MOVEMENT

The difference between the platform and the Hayes Double Leg Top Hops is the series of platforms to be jumped up on and off (see figure). The number of jumps is determined per set by the number of platforms.

SPEED-STRENGTH COACHING TIPS

A recommended workout program would be between 4-10 platforms and 2-5 series. Try, as a rule of thumb, to start low, and as the drills become more skillful, then add to the number of platforms and number of series. Another reminder is to keep the height of the platform between 12" and 18." The athlete wants to get a forceful drive off the top of each platform as well as the ground space between each platform. Start with an easy distance between each platform. As it becomes easier, move each platform a little further apart.

---

* Note: Coach Dean Hayes was the 1990 Goodwill Head Men's Track & Field Coach, the 1988 Men's Olympic Jump Coach and is presently the head Track & Field Coach for both men and women at Middle Tennessee State University.

DRILL 2: HAYES DOUBLE LEG IN THE HOLE HOPS

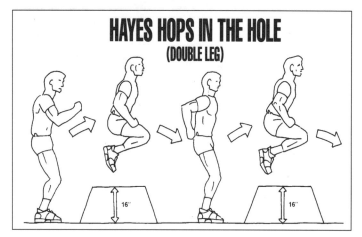

STARTING POSITION

Assume the same starting position as in the Hayes Double Leg in the Hole Top Hops.

THE ACTION OF THE MOVEMENT

Again, same as in the Hayes Double Leg Top Hops, the athlete will be moving over multi-platforms. The difference is this time instead of landing on the top of each platform, the athlete will land on the ground space between each platform (see Figure).

SPEED-STRENGTH CACHING TIPS

Recommended number of platforms should stay between 4-10 and 2-5 series. Remind the athlete that reaction speed between the ground recover time is to be kept at a minimum. Be aware of athletic form and technique.

DRILL 3: HAYES SINGLE LEG TOP HOPS

STARTING POSITION

Stand erect in a relaxed position (with either right or left knee up).

THE ACTION OF THE MOVEMENT

As in the Double Leg Top Hops, the difference will be only that one leg will be used at a time (see Figure). So if you use the right leg on the ground in one direction, use the left leg in the opposite.

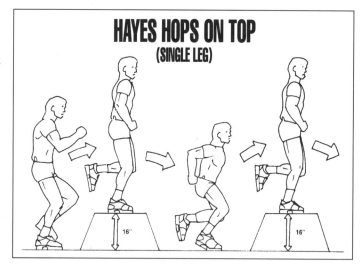

SPEED-STRENGTH COACHING TIP

The arms will be a great factor in the balancing of each reaction. Try to develop the arms' action as used in sprinting. Stay between 4-10 platforms and 2-5 series. These are excellent for the athlete who depends on quick reaction jumps and relies on the explosive jump in various sports of spontaneous reactions.

DRILL 4: HAYES SINGLE LEG IN THE HOLE HOPS

STARTING POSITION

The starting position is the same as in the Hayes Single Leg Top Hops.

THE ACTION OF THE MOVEMENT

Repeat as in the Hayes Double Leg in the Hole Hop; the difference will be only that one leg will be used at a time (see figure). The example is , again, right leg in one direction, left in the other.

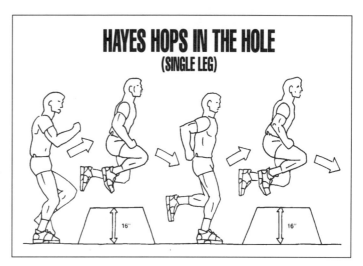

SPEED-STRENGTH COACHING TIPS

The distance between each platform should be minimal at first; then by repeating the movements, gradually move the platforms further apart from each other. Stay between 4-10 platforms and 2-5 series. These are excellent in the development in knee stability of cutting , darting and changing of direction. This drill is great for super reaction ability.

REACTION SPEED-STRENGTH SPRINTING DRILLS

These three running drills - bounds, running A's and skips -- integrated into the overall speed-strength training program will help in the development of sprint speed. By incorporating these three running drills into the development of speed, the athlete can identify wasted motion and movements that hinder his ability to obtain maximum running speed.

Each of these drills require the use of knee lift to arm action in teaching the athlete the correct and simplest technique in sprinting speed improvement.

BOUNDING DRILLS

Bounding is an excellent plyometric drill for developing speed, balance, coordination and agility. Bounding incorporates the skill of jumping and the mechanics of running all in one. The athletes' improvements are in stride length and stride frequency, two factors that make up running speed.

DRILL 1 - BOUNDS

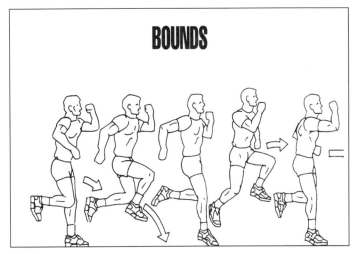

STARTING POSITION

Assume a good relaxed standing position at a defined starting line or point. You can either have both feet together or in a split leg position.

THE ACTION OF THE MOVEMENT

Bound as far as possible from one leg to the other, going up and forward on each leg. Land lightly on the balls of the feet and on to the toes. The center of gravity must be behind on each step and then pulled forward (see figure). The action is repeated several times for a given distance.

SPEED STRENGTH COACHING TIPS

By varying the workouts, the athlete can bound for distance, which is excellent for speed-strength, or take short, fast bounds which are good for speed explosion.

This is a very simple drill, but the pay-back is huge. Suggested distance, sets and repetitions are 20-60 yards, 2-4 sets and 2-6 repetitions per training day. Suggested number of days is 2-3 days per week.

DRILL 2: RUNNING A'S

STARTING POSITION

Assume a good relaxed standing position at a defined starting line or point. You can either have both feet together or in split leg position.

ACTION OF THE MOVEMENT

The running A's drill utilizes the maximum training movements for speed sprinting development. This drill is similar to the skip drill with the exception that the knee and arm action is at rapid movement speeds. Again, right arm to left leg action and left arm to right leg movement occurs in rapid-fire movement. The idea is to develop proper knee lift and arm action to promote faster reaction strength (see figure).

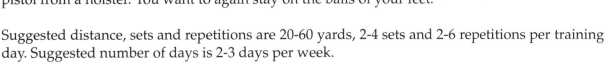

SPEED-STRENGTH COACHING TIPS

Make sure the knee lift is brought right above the belt line. Also, pump the arms slightly past the upper-torso side, a movement very similar to drawing a pistol from a holster. You want to again stay on the balls of your feet.

Suggested distance, sets and repetitions are 20-60 yards, 2-4 sets and 2-6 repetitions per training day. Suggested number of days is 2-3 days per week.

DRILL 3: SKIPS

STARTING POSITION

Assume a good relaxed standing position at a defined starting line or point. You either have both feet together or in a split leg position.

THE ACTION OF THE DRILL

In mastering the skip drill movement, the athlete should start with the walking position movement first. As the right leg touches the ground, the left arm should make a light touch to the right knee. As the left leg touches the ground, have the right arm lightly touch the left leg on the downward motion. Skipping incorporates rhythm, coordination and balance (see illustration). As the athlete advances form walking to slow running to the actual speed skip, he will be up on the balls of his feet, exerting smooth arm action.

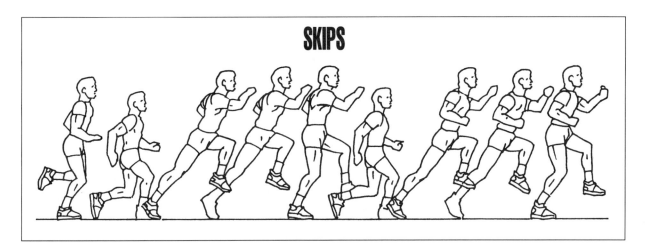

SPEED STRENGTH COACHING TIPS

For any athlete just starting, the skips allow for proper sprinting mechanism and proper balance awareness. Corrections of running form and techniques can be evaluated, and technique can be corrected.

Distance, sets and repetitions are 20-60 yards, 2-4 sets and 2-6 repetitions per day. Suggested number of days is 2-3 days per week.

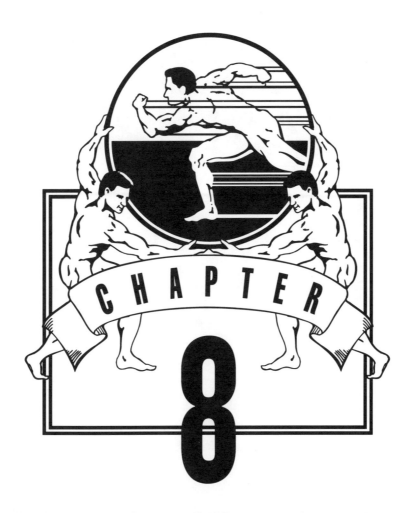

BALLISTICS-UPPER BODY EXPLOSIVENESS

"Whatever the mind of man can conceive and believe, it can be achieved."
Napoleon Hill
Author

BALLISTICS- UPPER BODY EXPLOSIVENESS

The use of the medicine ball throw stimulates the skills needed by an offensive lineman when pass blocking, a wide receiver catching a football, a running back being hit by a tackler or a defensive end pushing off a would-be blocker. In his book <u>Bounding to the Top</u> (1984), Coach Frank Costello recommends six to eight minutes of medicine ball training after every workout.

The athlete, trainee or football coach can review in this chapter different drills involving ballistic movements and select from eight different drills used in the development of speed-strength for football players. The medicine balls come in various sizes, weights and makes. What is best for the football player is determined by his level of strength. For standardized testing, the eight pound medicine ball would be ideal for the football player.

MEDICINE BALL THROWING DRILLS

The athlete should spend five to six minutes for the total number of exercises. The number of exercise drills incorporated on a training day should not be more than five or less than two. Any more drills or longer training sessions would decrease the overall explosive strength development.

Briefly, the idea of using the medicine ball throws and catches is important to teaching methods, form and techniques involved with catching a football. These drills allow the athlete to develop a feel for the ball and the ability to relax and concentrate upon impact with the thrown medicine ball.

Medicine ball throwing drills are best incorporated with a partner or by using a rebounder throw-back screen or by using the rubber medicine balls that bounce and can be thrown against a wall that will come back to the thrower. The following eight ballistic drills serve as examples of the types of medicine ball throws, ballistic push-ups and weight throws that may be used in a speed-strength training program.

DRILL 1: STANDING OVERHEAD THROW AND KNEELING

OVERHEAD THROW

STARTING POSITION

Start by placing the feet shoulder width apart. Grip the ball with both hands and bring the ball back as far as possible over the head (Figure 128).

THE ACTION OF THE MOVEMENT

Keep the arms bent at a ninety degree angle at the elbows. The stretch occurring in the shoulders, chest, latissimus dorsi and leg muscles helps the athlete to know when to step forward with either leg and at the same time pull the elbows forward and throw the ball (Figure 129).

SPEED-STRENGTH COACHING TIPS.

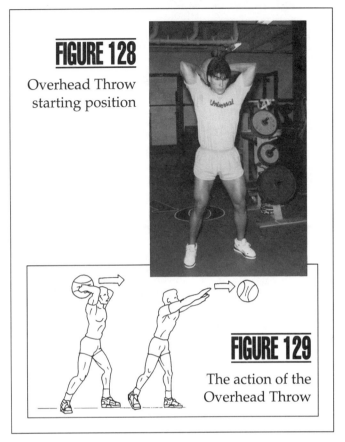

FIGURE 128
Overhead Throw starting position

FIGURE 129
The action of the Overhead Throw

Remind the athlete to grip the ball firmly and follow through with each throw. Distance should vary according to the strength level of each player and weight of the medicine balls.

KNEELING OVERHAND THROW

The procedure for this throw is the same as the standing overhead throw, except the athlete is on his knees. This throwing exercise requires strength in the upper and lower back. Be sure to follow through after releasing the ball.

DRILL 2: STANDING SIDE THROW

STARTING POSITION.

The starting procedure is also the same for this drill as for the overhead throws.

THE ACTION OF THE MOVEMENT.

As the ball is being brought back to one side, have the athlete keep it away from the body. As the ball is being thrown back, rotate the hips forward to get a good stretch in the entire left side of the body (Figure 130).

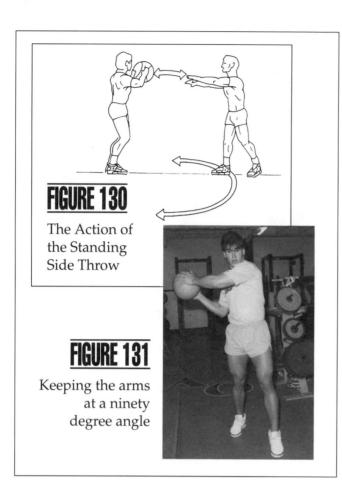

FIGURE 130

The Action of the Standing Side Throw

FIGURE 131

Keeping the arms at a ninety degree angle

SPEED-STRENGTH COACHING TIPS

Remember to keep the ninety degree angle in the arms. Finish as in the overhead throw. Muscles in the rectus abdominis and external oblique on the opposite of the throwing side are being worked, as well as the muscles used in the overhead throws (Figure 131).

DRILL 3: TWO-HAND CHEST THROW

STARTING POSITION

The starting procedure is also the same as the overhead, except the throw is from the chest (Figure 132).

THE ACTION OF THE MOVEMENT

As the ball is being brought back to the chest, keep the elbows even at shoulder level. Step forward with either leg, and push the throw through to full release and follow through. Muscles being worked are those of the chest, shoulders, legs and arms.

SPEED-STRENGTH COACHING TIPS

This is an excellent drill for teaching shoulder, arm and chest explosion, as well as catching or receiving skills used by receivers.

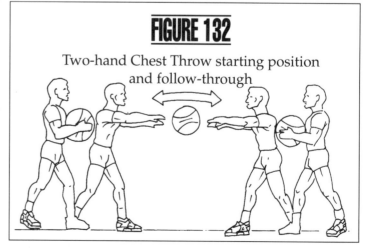

FIGURE 132

Two-hand Chest Throw starting position and follow-through

DRILL 4: SIT-UP THROW AND SIT-UP LONG THROW

STARTING POSITION

Assume the bent knee, sit-up position (Figure 133).

THE ACTION OF THE MOVEMENT

The athlete is to throw the ball as he is raising upward and forward. Figure 133A illustrates the position of the legs so that the balance for the throwing motion can occur. The position of the ball is similar to that of the overhead throw. Remember to follow through upon release.

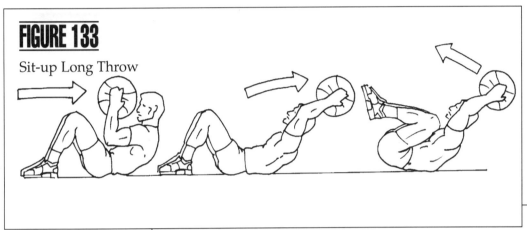

FIGURE 133
Sit-up Long Throw

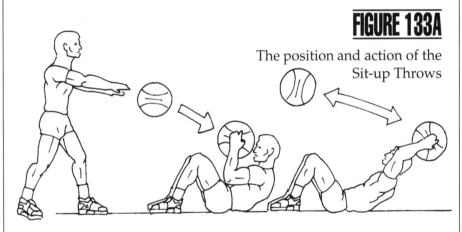

FIGURE 133A
The position and action of the Sit-up Throws

SPEED-STRENGTH COACHING TIPS

This is an excellent exercise for the mid-section. It is also a good drill to use with a teammate or training partner for a combination exercise for throwing and stomach work. Also, by implementing the sit-up long-throw, the distance will be greater. This drill is excellent for the hip flexion-development and coordination.

DRILL 5: UNDERHAND/BACK OVERHEAD THROW

STARTING POSITION

Assume the standing athletic position with feet shoulder width apart. Reversing the movement of action, this time the movement is from front to back (Figure 134).

THE ACTION OF THE MOVEMENT

Keep the ball out front and away from the body. Assume a squat position about three-fourths of the way down. The action will be a sweeping movement of up and over the head (Figure 135).

SPEED-STRENGTH COACHING TIPS

Release of the ball will occur at the point of optimal stretching of the shoulders, back, arms and legs. This is an excellent drill for offensive lineman because football calls for the force of driving the arms and hands upwards.

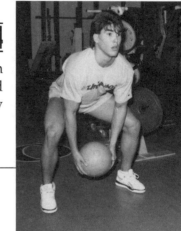

FIGURE 134

Starting position of the Underhand Throw

FIGURE 135

The action of a sweeping movement

DRILL 6: BENCH PRESS THROW

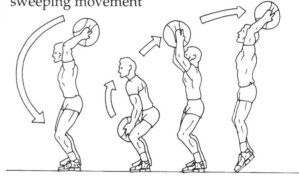

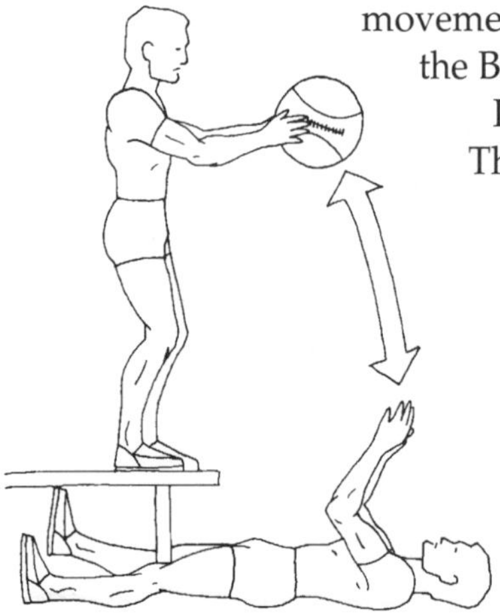

FIGURE 136

Starting position and action movement in the Bench Press Throw

STARTING POSITION

Assume the position of having the athlete lie down on his back with the arms extended upward and ready to catch the ball. This exercise should help a football player catch the ball and improve the punching or striking speed-strength movement (Figure 136).

THE ACTION OF THE MOVEMENT

Take a position lying on the floor; have the workout partner stand above the supine (on back) player. The athlete standing above the player will drop the ball to the center position on the chest. The player is prepared to catch the ball and immediately throw the ball back to the standing player. This action will allow the player to use short, explosive arm and chest movements with no loading (pulling back) for the release (Figure 136).

SPEED-STRENGTH COACHING TIPS

The use of hands required of the offensive line makes this drill one that should be employed time and time again. Because the athlete is lying on the floor, the elbows cannot extend past the sides. The defensive players make use of the quick, explosive force that is generated.

DRILL 7: PRESS THROW

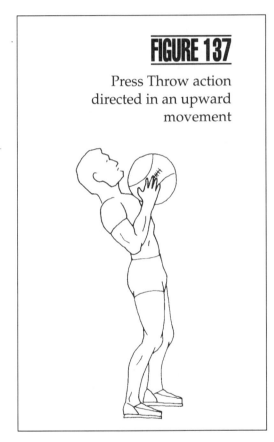

FIGURE 137

Press Throw action directed in an upward movement

STARTING POSITION

Assume a shoulder width standing position (Figure 137). The head and shoulders are slightly tilted backward.

THE ACTION OF THE MOVEMENT

Grip the ball with both hands. The head will be looking upward and will allow the back and hip position to prepare for the throwing motion. Squeeze and extend the arms through the throw as the ball travels in an upward direction and then prepare to make the catch (Figure 137).

SPEED-STRENGTH COACHING TIPS

This exercise is an excellent one for all football positions and is outstanding for eye-hand coordination, as well as for developing the ability to keep the opponent at arms' length, a distinction so important in keeping the blocker or tackler away from the body. Here the athlete can perform a drill that does not require a partner and can fully use his available training time by not having to retrieve the thrown ball.

BALLISTIC PUSH-UP

The ballistic push-up incorporates speed-strength training components and principles of upper body explosion in a training movement. The use of the hands (arm and shoulder explosion) by the offensive line exemplifies the need for exercises and strength movements that can improve the speed and strength of this offensive skill.

Not to be forgotten is the use of hands (arm-shoulder use) by the defensive players. The skills used by the defensive players against the run and when rushing the passer are the opposite of

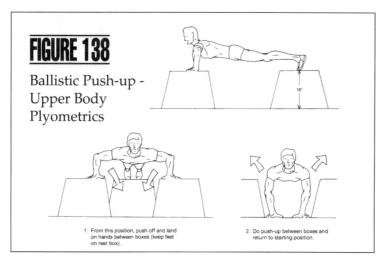

FIGURE 138

Ballistic Push-up - Upper Body Plyometrics

the offensive player whose job is to be able to run, block and pass protect against the defensive charge. This is an excellent exercise which promotes the use of hands in football skill techniques (Figure 138).

DRILL 8: BALLISTIC PUSH-UP

STARTING POSITION

Assume the position with arms separated and feet together planted on top of the platforms in a prone position with weight of the body separated equally at each point (Figure 139).

THE ACTION OF THE MOVEMENT

Lower the body by bending the arms and dropping down between the two platforms (Figure 140). To start the push-up, repeat the downward push and explode upward by pushing off the floor with both arms and shoulders.

SPEED-STRENGTH COACHING TIPS

This exercise begins with the regular push-up drill. After the regular push-ups are completed, have the football player start off with a minimum platform and gradually work up to a maximum height of no more than eighteen inches. Remind the players to concentrate on exploding off the floor.

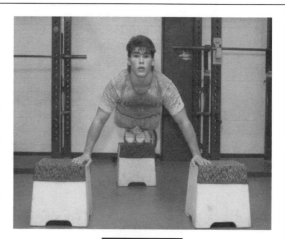

FIGURE 139

Starting position of the Ballistic Push-up

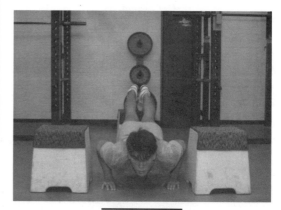

FIGURE 140

Downward action of the Drop Between the Two Platforms

WEIGHT THROWS

One area that can be extremely helpful to the high school football athlete is the use of weight implements, primarily those used in track and field--the shot put, discus, hammer, javelin and weight throw. Any of these weight events are excellent supplements. However, it is not mandatory to include weight throwing to have a successful program. However, what could make throws so valuable to the football player is the opportunity to practice developing speed and strength in a sporting event that requires the athlete to compete, concentrate and employ different coordinations.

The use of weight lifting exercises and weight training alone develops only one dimension of speed-strength. By incorporating the use of ballistic drills of upper body explosiveness--medicine ball throwing, ballistic push-ups and weight throws--the improved overall development moves the player to a greater level of speed-strength. The use of ballistic drills allows the athlete to improve the total speed-strength potential (Figure 141).

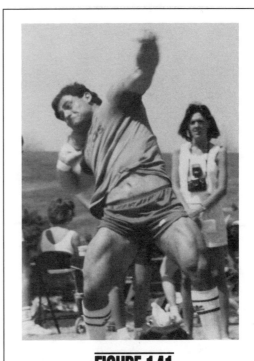

FIGURE 141

Use of the Shot-put as a different kind of weight throw movement

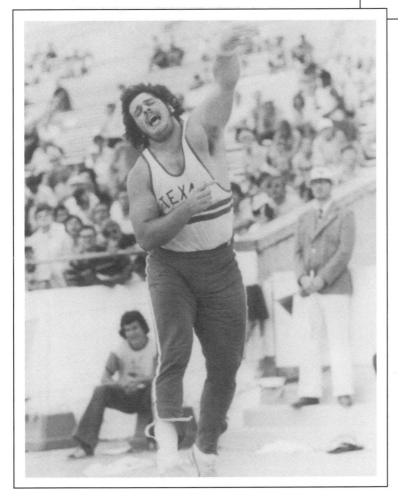

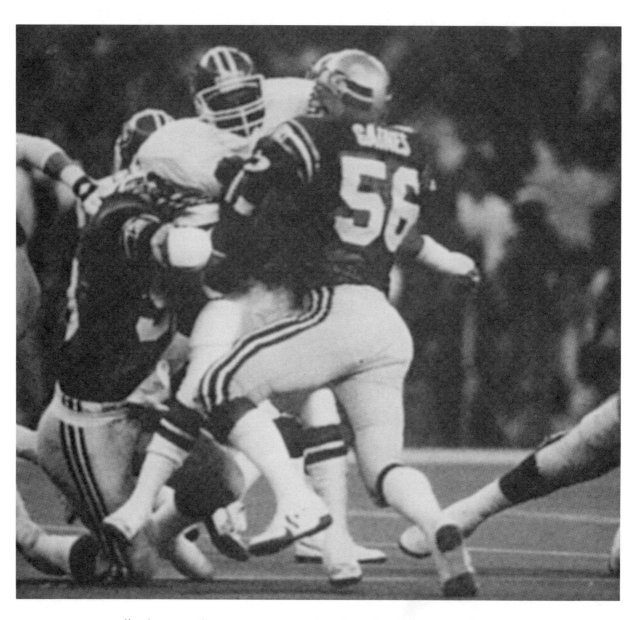

"The only way to acheive is to practice."
E. J. "Doc" Kreis

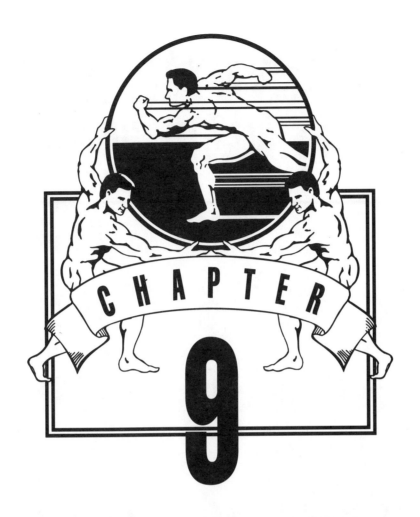

CHAPTER 9

EVALUATION AND TESTING OF SPEED-STRENGTH TRAINING

"Before I get in the ring, I'd have already won or lost it out on the road. The real part is won or lost somewhere far away from witnesses - behind the lines, in the gym and out there on the road before I dance under those lights."
Muhammad Ali
Professional Boxer

EVALUATION AND TESTING OF SPEED-STRENGTH TRAINING

There is no appropriate substitute for evaluation and testing. What can be implemented from a knowledge of results far outweighs the approach of "Let's wait and see what happens." Succeeding because of a legitimate plan of action leads to reduction of errors and mistakes in a training program.

WHEN TO EVALUATE

The annual training cycle for high school football players in speed-strength training has three evaluation and testing times. Running, reaction-speed, strength, jumping and throwing should be the main movements evaluated and tested.

The three main evaluation and testing times are:

1. At the end of the general preparatory period--preparatory phase--week seven to the first week in March;

2. At the end of the specific preparatory period--preparatory phase--week nine to the third week in May;

3. At the end of the pre-competitive period--competitive period, week six to the second week in July (See Chapter 2, page 12, Table 2 for Speed-Strength Training Program for High School Football).

A coach may want to include an optional fourth or fifth evaluation and testing time either during the football season or shortly afterward. To incorporate an optional fourth or fifth evaluation and testing time, the suggested time would be the second or third week in November or the first or second week in January.

For incoming freshmen, the suggested initial evaluation and testing time would be in late January or late May, just after the third evaluation and testing period. This approach allows the coach to use the last weeks in May as an orientation period for the new football players and also would allow for a six-week working cycle before re-evaluation and testing.

RUNNING RACES

The purpose of evaluation and testing in the running races is to help the coach, trainer or athlete distinguish between the following: (1) quick speed, (2) running speed, (3) strength speed and (4) endurance speed, all of which are recorded to the nearest hundredth of a second. The following are examples of the four kinds of running races that should be evaluated and tested:

Race 1   40-yard dash--quick start and acceleration of speed--Run one each;

Race 2   60-yard dash--running speed to maintain the starting point and pickup of acceleration in a longer sprint--Run one each;

Race 3   100-yard dash--speed generated and maintained over quick speed and speed-strength--Run one each;

Race 4   880-yard run--endurance speed--tests mental toughness of a football player--Run one each.

By evaluating and testing the football players in these running races, the football coach or trainer can better evaluate the running talent of his players. For some of the players, the times will represent a beginning reference point. Regardless of how big or small the athlete may be, the recorded facts concerning him (how quick, fast, strong and tough in running) may give a little more insight concerning the best possible position for the young football player. This approach also represents a good way to evaluate the talent of both running and attitude (Tables 9 and 10).

TABLE 9

Drills of Running Speed
Individual Sheet

Name	Body Weight	40-Yd. Dash	60 Yd. Dash	100 Yd. Dash	880 Yd Dash
Pretest					
Protest					

Time _____   Time _____
Month Day Year   Month Day Year

TABLE 10

Running Speed
Master Record

Test Period _____

Time of Day _____   Month Day Year _____

Name	Body Weight	40-Yd. Dash	60 Yd. Dash	100 Yd. Dash	880 Yd Dash
1					
2					
3					
4					
5					
6					

RACES 1, 2, 3: 40-, 60-, AND 100-YARD DASHES

STARTING POSITION

Allow the football player to use a starting position that will give him the greatest amount of force off the starting line. This can either be a one-arm or two-arm track starting stance. The same kind of stance is used for each of the three races.

THE ACTION OF THE RACE

The football player wants to generate quick and fast speed that will allow him to cover the desired distance in the least amount of time.

SPEED-STRENGTH COACHING TIPS

Remind the athletes to run through the finish line. Also, remind them not to worry for the present about form or technique, but to run all-out. This is also a good time to demonstrate proper warm-up routines before racing. Record the time for each player as he runs his races. The timers will start their clocks when the athlete makes his "first movement." Times are recorded to the nearest hundredth of a second.

RACE 4: 880-YARD RUN

STARTING POSITION

Players can be divided into specialty groups. If using a running track, the starting position is taken at the starting line, which will also be the finish line (if one lap is 440 yards).

THE ACTION OF THE RUN

The two-lap distance for endurance speed is a test (pre and post) to help develop mental toughness in the football player. The purpose for this running action is to enable the athlete to endure a distance farther than he would be asked to run on a football field.

SPEED-STRENGTH COACHING TIPS

Evaluation and testing of football players provide a solid data base which can be used to develop progressive speed and strength in the players. The amount of gain during a training cycle or period is clearly identified, recorded and used as a tool of evaluation for speed-strength training. Remember that all the races should be timed, beginning with the first movement of the athlete.

REACTION-SPEED DRILLS

Evaluation and testing of reaction-speed drills will assist the trainer or football coach in determining speed-strength of the football player (Tables 11 and 12). *The ability to display "quick feet" is of utmost importance.*

Following are the procedures and methods to be used for evaluating reaction-speed drills.

TABLE 11

Reaction Drills of Speed-Strength
Master Record

Time of Day				Month Day Year
Name	Body Weight	Line Touch	Figure Eight	Four Corner
1				
2				

TABLE 12

Reaction Drills of Speed-Strength
Individual Sheet

Time				Time			
Month Day Year				Month Day Year			
Name	Body Weight	Line Touch	Figure Eight	Four Corner			
Pretest							
Protest							

DRILL 1: LINE TOUCH

STARTING POSITION

The football player is positioned in the middle position between the two lines that will be touched (Figure 142). The starting direction to be followed by the player has already been decided.

THE ACTION OF THE DRILL

The time starts with the first movement of the player. The player positions himself in the center of the ten-yard distance. Then he is told to stay low and move as quickly and as fast as possible. The ten-yard distance is covered by touching one side and then the other side one time each. The reaction speed to the final touch is a ten-yard sprint past the finishing point (Figure 142).

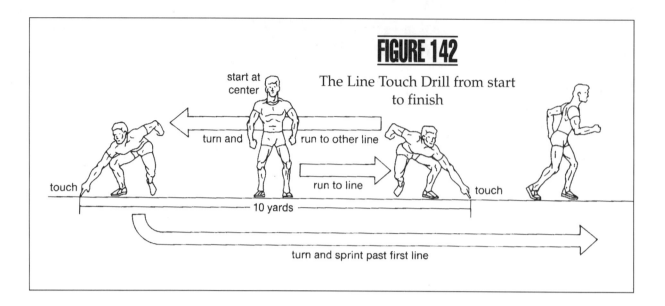

FIGURE 142

The Line Touch Drill from start to finish

SPEED-STRENGTH COACHING TIPS

If the coach does not have enough personnel to see that each player touches each line, he may have the player pick up and deliver two-by-four inch wooden blocks, instead of hand touching the lines. Remind the athletes to not cross their feet, stay low and drive off each line touch. Record two completed efforts (side-to-side reaction two times).

DRILL 2: FIGURE EIGHT

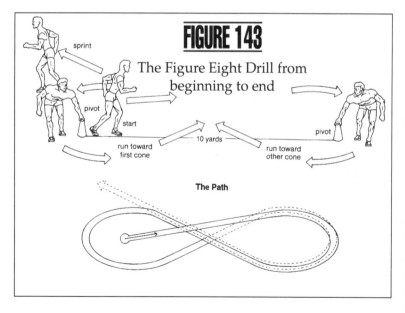

FIGURE 143

The Figure Eight Drill from beginning to end

STARTING POSITION

The football player is positioned at the starting line. The athlete can choose any kind of starting stance. (Figure 143).

THE ACTION OF THE RACE

The race requires the player to cover the required distance in the least amount of time. The player must pivot and turn around each of the two cones placed ten yards apart. The player drives off the starting line and sprints to the first cone, turns and pivots and drives to the starting cone. Again, he pivots and turns (he may place his hands down) and drives back to the first cone, repeats, and then sprints past the starting line), which is now the finish line (Figure 143).

SPEED-STRENGTH COACHING TIPS

This is a more difficult reaction-speed drill. It is a good idea to have the athletes perform a practice run for this drill. The equipment used includes plastic traffic cones. Remind the athlete to place the hand down and pivot around each turn as quickly as possible. Record two completed cycles. The coach looks for explosive starts, good acceleration, balance and coordination in this race.

DRILL 3: FOUR CORNER

STARTING POSITION

The football player takes a standing position at the starting line. The stance used is the player's choice (Figure 144).

THE ACTION OF THE DRILL

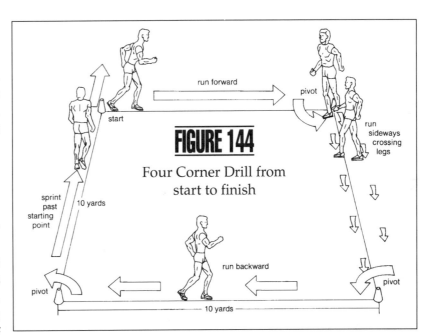

FIGURE 144

Four Corner Drill from start to finish

The ultimate for reaction-speed is the four-corner drill. The athlete assumes his starting position and moves toward the cone markers. The starting movement is a straight run. At the point of approaching the first cone, the pivot is made inward, and the movement is now a crossing-leg movement called <u>carrioca</u>. Approaching the second cone, the player again pivots to the inside and then runs backwards (back peddling) to the third corner. The pivot at the third cone is again approached with an inward movement and drive. The movement after the inside pivot at the third cone is a sprint through the fourth and finishing cone (Figure 144).

SPEED-STRENGTH COACHING TIPS

The four-corner is the ultimate for speed-strength running drills; it has it all. The football coach or trainer should discuss the importance of reaction-speed and the transfer values that the four-corner drill provides. Two complete cycles are recorded for each player. Remind the players to always pivot when making the turns at cones 1, 2 and 3.

STRENGTH

The purpose for evaluating and testing strength is to help the football coach identify the level of strength that each of his players possesses. Determining the player's level, starting point and strength condition allows the coach to incorporate an individualized speed-strength training program to benefit all his football players. The proper speed-strength program will help develop the basic techniques of football--blocking, running, throwing and catching (Table 13).

After the initial evaluation and testing, the football coach has an opportunity to evaluate what has been accomplished from the starting point of the speed-strength training program (Table 14). The following exercises of strength should be evaluated and tested:

Exercise 1. Chin-ups--as many as possible

Exercise 2. Dips--as many as possible

Exercise 3. Bench press--maximum attempts

Exercise 4. Back squat--maximum attempts

Exercise 5. Power clean--maximum attempts

Exercise 6. Military press--maximum attempts (standing position).

TABLE 13

Strength Record

Time _____ Time _____
Month Day Year   Month Day Year

Name _____
Body Weight _____
Football Position _____

Record Best Efforts

	Pre	Post	Pre	Post	Pre	Post
Back Squat						
Military Press						
Dip (most done in succession)						
Chin-up (most done in succession)						

TABLE 14

Master Sheet for Coach
Speed-Strength Best Man Lifted

Time _____
Month Day Year

Name	Bench Press	Front Squat	Back Squat	Power Clean	C&J J&S	Dips	Chin-ups	Vertical Jumps	Stading Long Jump	Power snatch

Note: C & J = Clean & Jerk
J & S = Jerk from Stand
(Dip and Chin-ups = most that can be done without stopping)

Maximum attempts should reflect a good effort, but not one that is an all-out, gut-busting attempt where the athlete forsakes good form and technique (Table 15).

This is a very important testing process. The introduction by the coach will include discussion about the attitude necessary for lifters just starting out who have never been exposed to a speed-strength lifting program. The coach needs to make it loud and clear that no lift should be attempted where the technique and method are ignored. This keeps the young athlete from foolishly attempting more than he really can lift; plus the coach should restate that the evaluation and testing are for the purpose of establishing a starting point for new athletes and a reevaluation of the players already in the program.

The testing procedure and methods of testing should follow the exercise description as presented in Chapters 3, 4 & 5 concerning the use of proper technique, form and method.

TABLE 15
Strength Record Board

Time: Month ___ Day ___ Year ___

Weight Class	Back Squat	Front Squat	Bench Press	Power Clean	Power Snatch	Clean & Jerk	Dips	Chin-ups
109	Name/Weight							
114								
123								
132								
148								
155								
168								
181								
198								
220								
242								
275								
Super Heavy								

Note: This same style of record board can be mounted on any wall or walls in the weight room or hallways or entrance.

JUMPING

The purpose of the jumping evaluation and testing is to help the trainer or football coach evaluate the "explosive leg strength" of his football players and their ability to incorporate and transfer the skill developed in football. The three different jumps help measure the following:
(1) vertical jump (VJ)--quick jumping reaction, (2) standing long jump (SLJ)--strength and jumping reaction and (3) triple long jump (TLJ)--the distance and jumping reaction. This gives some measure of vertical and horizontal jumping explosiveness and starting strength. Evaluation and testing consist of: (1) vertical jump--measure the height of a vertical jump--two attempts, (2) standing long jump--measure for length of a single horizontal jump--two attempts and (3) standing triple jump--three jump series measuring distance--two attempts (Tables 16 and 17).

The evaluation and testing allow for a review of the football player's improvement in jumping.

Listed are the procedures and methods for evaluating and testing the jumps. For further information of the training jumps, refer to Chapter 7 on plyometrics.

TABLE 17
Jumping Max- Master Record

	Time of day			Month Day Year	
	Name	Body Weight	Vertical Jump	Standing Long Jump	Starting Triple Jump
1					
2					
3					
4					
5					
6					
7					
8					

Note: Place and asterisk (*) in area of new PR.

TABLE 16
Jumping Max

	Time of day			Month Day Year	
	Name	Body Weight	Vertical Jump	Standing Long Jump	Starting Triple Jump
Pretest					
Protest					
Posttest					

Difference of Jumps _____ (+ or - distance) circle one

Note: Place and asterisk (*) in area of new PR.

DRILL 1: VERTICAL JUMP

STARTING POSITION

The athlete approaches the marking boards. He raises his arm to full extension and places his fingers against the board so that a mark can be left for marking (Figure 145).

THE ACTION OF THE JUMP

The athlete positions himself to jump as high as possible, leaving his mark to be measured and recorded. The athlete has both feet in the suited jumping stance. No movement of either foot (no stepping back, either) is allowed before the jump is completed. Record the highest of two jumps (Figure 146).

SPEED-STRENGTH COACHING TIPS

The chalk used for marking can be the same chalk used in lifting.

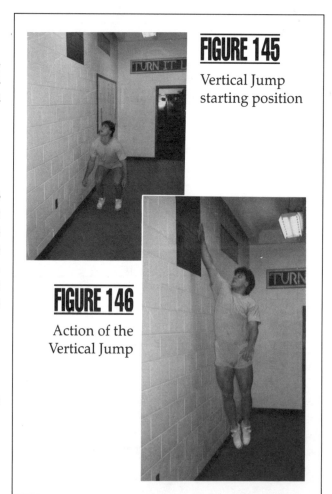

FIGURE 145
Vertical Jump starting position

FIGURE 146
Action of the Vertical Jump

DRILL 2: STANDING LONG JUMP

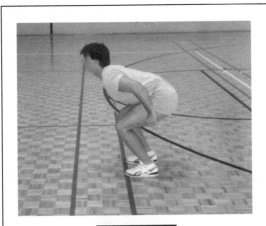

FIGURE 147
Standing Long Jump starting position

STARTING POSITION

The athlete takes a position close to the starting line (Figure 147).

THE ACTION OF THE JUMP

Once the athlete jumps and lands feet first, neither foot can move. For the long jump to be recorded, the athlete must "stick" the jump. This test allows two jumps.

SPEED-STRENGTH COACHING TIPS

This drill encourages football players to increase flexibility and dexterity.
Remind the athlete that he must "stick" the jump--cannot move either of his feet upon landing. Also, remind the players to turn their toes slightly in preparing to leap.

DRILL 3: STANDING TRIPLE JUMP

STARTING POSITION

The same rules apply as in the long jump, except one must do three consecutive jumps.

THE ACTION OF THE JUMP

This test measures the length of the starting to finishing jump (test is two triple jumps). This test is achieved with three consecutive jumps. Use the same techniques and form that are displayed in the standing long jump. Also, the use of the arms coordinated with the legs improves the forward momentum of the entire body.

SPEED-STRENGTH COACHING TIPS

Remind the football players to jump as far as possible on each of the three jumps. The total distance is then recorded. Stress that each jump is as important as the other. This test is a combination of the vertical and standing long jump and measures endurance jumping and speed-strength.

MEDICINE BALL THROWS

The purpose of medicine ball throwing tests is to help measure upper-body explosive strength in the football player.

The evaluation and testing of throwing consist of the following medicine ball drills: (1) seated long throw for distance, (2) standing long throw for distance and (3) standing backward long throw for distance. An eight-pound medicine ball is used. Post-testing allows the coach to evaluate the amount of upper-body explosive, starting and absolute strength that has been transferred to the skill of throwing (Tables 18 and 19).

Following are three examples of throwing tests. For further information on throwing, refer to Chapter 8 on ballistics.

TABLE 18

Throwing Maximum Distance
Individual Sheet

Time _____ Month Day Year _____

Name	Seated Long Throw	Standing Long Throw	Standing Back Overhead Throw
Pretest			
Protest			

Note: Place an asterisk (*) in the area of new PR.

TABLE 19

Throwing Maximum Distance
Individual Sheet

Time _____ Month Day Year _____

Name	Seated Long Throw		Standing Long Throw		Standing Backwards Throw	
	Pre	Post	Pre	Post	Pre	Post
1						
2						
3						
4						
5						
6						
7						
8						

Note: Place an asterisk (*) in the area of new PR.
Pre = Pretest
Post = Postest

DRILL 1: SEATED LONG THROW

STARTED POSITION

The athlete positions himself in a seated position on the throwing surface, keeping heels and feet behind the line (Figure 148).

THE ACTION OF THE THROW

Placing the medicine ball behind the head, the athlete attempts to project the ball forward in an explosive manner as far as possible. The longest of two attempts is recorded.

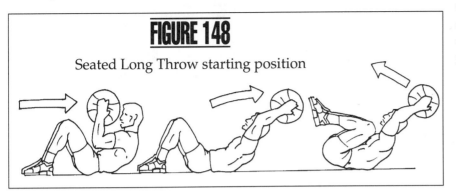

FIGURE 148

Seated Long Throw starting position

SPEED-STRENGTH COACHING TIPS

This test allows the coach to measure movement of the upper body's ballistic speed-strength. Make sure that a warm-up routine of practice throws between 4-8 in preparation of a measured attempt is incorporated.

DRILL 2: STANDING LONG THROW

STARTING POSITION.

The athlete positions himself in a standing position on the throwing surface, keeping heels and feet behind the line.

THE ACTION OF THE THROW

Placing the medicine ball behind his head, the athlete projects the ball forward in an explosive manner to achieve the greatest distance. The longest of two attempts is recorded (Figure 149).

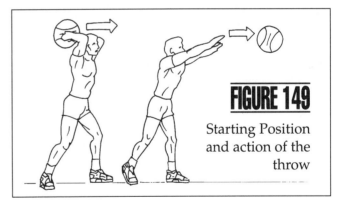

FIGURE 149

Starting Position and action of the throw

SPEED-STRENGTH COACHING TIPS

This is an excellent exercise to evaluate a transfer of coordination of speed-strength incorporating the total body's coordination. Make sure the medicine balls are dry and the player uses both hands on the ball for the throw.

DRILL 3: STANDING BACK OVERHEAD LONG THROW

STARTING POSITION

The athlete positions himself as close to the starting line as possible without stepping on or over it (foul).

THE ACTION OF THE THROW

Standing on the throwing surface, the athlete throws the medicine ball backward and over the body. Two attempts are required for recorded measure (Figure 150).

SPEED-STRENGTH COACHING TIPS

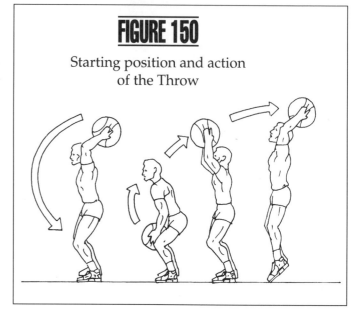

FIGURE 150

Starting position and action of the Throw

This is a more difficult throwing drill. It requires a higher degree of balance and athletic skill. Remind the players to not step over the line.

BODY MEASUREMENTS

Recording body measurements is one of the oldest methods utilized for gathering information on the muscle development of athletes. Body measurements are important for the following reasons:

1. Measurements of the football player's body help the coach keep updated information on the size of his athletes and also will serve as a check and balance of muscle size improvements.

2. Measurements taken one month and retaken every four months will help the coach appraise the progress or digression of his players. Example: (a) first of January--measurements taken, (b) first of April--measure-ments taken and (c) first of August--measurements taken (Table 20).

TABLE 20

Personal Profile
Measurements

First Name ____ Last Name ____ Time of day ____ Month Day Year
Age ____ Date of Birth ____ Football Position ____

A. Neck ____
B. Chest ____
C. Thighs ____ Right ____ Left
D. Arms ____ Right ____ Left
E. Shoulders ____
F. Waist ____
G. Calves ____ Right ____ Left
Weight ____
Height ____

3. Measurements tell the coach if the program of training is working.

4. Method of measurement should be consistent.

5. Invest is a good tape measure that will ensure consistent measurements. A steel tape is the best investment.

6. Be consistent in how the measurements are recorded.

SELF-EVALUATION TRAINING JOURNAL

Records of all athletes should be kept by the football coach. Just as important is a self-evaluation training journal which should be kept by each athlete. In the seminar by Coach Gregory Goldstein, formerly of the Soviet Union coaching staff, he made the point that an athlete who does not bring his lifting journal to practice should immediately be sent home and not allowed to practice that day. The coach may allow the football players to carry the self-evaluation journals home, but it is better to have a filing shelf or designated area in the facility.

By keeping his own journal and noting updates with each workout, each athlete can monitor his progress and is more motivated to succeed in his speed-strength training. The self-evaluation training journal serves to point out the good training days and what made them good and also point out weak days and when they occurred. The self-evaluation training journal also notes one's personal records (PR's) and what new goals he is training to achieve. The coach can refer to his own records while reviewing the football player's journal and make helpful suggestions with this improved insight into the athlete's thinking and motivating factors (Table 21).

TABLE 21

Self-Evaluation Training Journal

First Name _____ Last Name _____ Phone _____

Day of Week _____ Month _____ Day _____ Year _____

Workout Week _____ and _____ Body Weight _____
Day of Week

Starting Time _____

Finishing Time _____

Warm-up Routine

Notes:

Personal Records (PRs) in:

Personal Training Record

Date _____ Time _____ Training

Body weight before training _____ After it _____

Self-feeling before training _____

During the time of training _____

After training _____

Notions of the coach _____

Number of exercises in order	Name of exercise	Volume and intensity	Zone S = Small M = Medium B = Big	Total number of Repetitions

Total Reps _____

Personal Training Record

Date: Monday - example Time: Non-competitive Training

Body weight before training _____ After it _____

Self-feeling before training _____

During the time of training _____

After training _____

Notions of the coach _____

Number of exercises in order	Name of exercise	Volume and intensity	Zone S = Small M = Medium B = Big	Total number of Repetitions
*	Warm-up Routine			
	1. One-legged Squat	3 sets × 6 reps		
	2. Glute Ham Raises	3 sets × 8 reps		
	3. Shoulder Flexers	3 sets × 10 reps		
	4. Standing Long Jump	1 set × 9 reps		
1.	Clean Pull	$\frac{50}{4}$ 2 $\frac{60}{4}$ $\frac{70}{3}$ $\frac{80}{3}$ 2	B	21
2.	Snatch	$\frac{55}{4}$ $\frac{60}{3}$ 2 $\frac{70}{4}$ 2	M	18
3.	Power Clean	$\frac{60}{5}$ $\frac{65}{5}$ 2	S	15
4.	Jerk from Rack	$\frac{50}{5}$ 2 $\frac{55}{5}$ $\frac{60}{5}$	S	20
5.	Back Squat	$\frac{50}{5}$ $\frac{55}{4}$ $\frac{60}{5}$ 3	S	24
6.	Bench Press	$\frac{50}{5}$ $\frac{60}{4}$ $\frac{70}{5}$ 2 $\frac{75}{5}$ 2	M	29
7.	Chin-ups	3 sets × 6 reps		
8.	Plyometrics - Hayes Hops			
	1. Double on Top	3 series × 8 platforms		
	2. Double in Hole	" "		
	3. Single on Top	" "		
	4. Single in Hole	" "		
9.	Ballistics - Standing Drills			
	1. Two Hand Chest Throw	3 sets × 8 reps		
	2. Standing Overhead Throw	" "		
10.	Weighted Sit-ups	$\frac{25\ lbs}{10\ reps}$ 3 sets		
*	Relaxation and Flexibility			
	1. Chin-up Pull Downs	3 × 8 seconds		
	2. Side to Side	3 × 6 reps		
	3. Split Squat Stretch	3 × 5 reps		

Total Reps ___127___

Personal Training Record

Date: __Tuesday - example__   Time: _____   Training

Body weight before training _____   After it _____

Self-feeling before training _____

During the time of training _____

After training _____

Notions of the coach _____

Number of exercises in order	Name of exercise	Volume and intensity	Zone S = Small M = Medium B = Big	Total number of Repetitions
*	Warm-up Routine			
	1. One-legged Squat	3 sets x 6 reps		
	2. Glute Ham Raises	3 sets x 8 reps		
	3. Shoulder Flexers	3 sets x 10 reps		
	4. Standing Long Jump	1 set x 9 reps		
1.	Snatch Pull	$\frac{50}{5}$ $\frac{60}{4}$ 2 $\frac{65}{4}$ $\frac{70}{4}$ 2	M	25
2.	Split Snatch	$\frac{50}{4}$ $\frac{55}{3}$ $\frac{60}{4}$ 3	S	19
3.	Clean and Jerk	$\frac{60}{4}$ $\frac{70}{3}$ 2 $\frac{80}{3}$ $\frac{85}{2}$ 3	B	19
4.	Front Squat	$\frac{55}{5}$ $\frac{65}{4}$ $\frac{70}{5}$ 2	M	19
5.	Closed Grip Bench Press	$\frac{50}{5}$ $\frac{60}{4}$ 4	S	21
6.	Dips	$\frac{25 \text{ lbs}}{6}$ 4		
7.	Plyometrics - Speed Strength Running Drills			
	1. Skips	60 yds. x 4 reps		
	2. Bounds	60 yds. x 4 reps		
	3. Running A's	60 yds. x 4 reps		
8.	Ballistics - Floor Drills			
	1. Kneeling Overhead Throw	3 sets x 8 reps		
	2. Sit-up Throw	3 sets x 8 reps		
9.	Weighted Sit-ups	$\frac{25 \text{ lbs.}}{10}$ 3		
*	Relaxation and Flexibility			
	1. Chin-up Pull Downs	3 x 8 seconds		
	2. Side to Side	3 x 6 reps		
	3. Split Squat Stretch	3 x 5 reps		

Total Reps ___103___

Personal Training Record

Date __Thursday-example__ Time _____ Training

Body weight before training _____ After it _____

Self-feeling before training _____

During the time of training _____

After training _____

Notions of the coach _____

Number of exercises in order	Name of exercise	Volume and intensity	Zone S = Small M = Medium B = Big	Total number of Repetitions
*	Warm-up Routine			
	1. One-legged Squat	3 sets x 6 reps		
	2. Glute Ham Raises	3 sets x 8 reps		
	3. Shoulder Flexers	3 sets x 10 reps		
	4. Standing Long Jump	1 set x 9 reps		
1.	Clean Pull	$\frac{55}{4}$ $\frac{65}{4}$ $\frac{75}{3}$ $\frac{85}{3}$ 4	B	23
2.	Snatch	$\frac{55}{4}$ $\frac{60}{3}$ $\frac{65}{3}$ 2 $\frac{75}{4}$ 2	M	21
3.	Power Clean	$\frac{55}{4}$ 2 $\frac{65}{4}$ $\frac{75}{4}$ 3	M	24
4.	Jerk from Rack	$\frac{55}{4}$ $\frac{60}{4}$ $\frac{70}{3}$ $\frac{75}{3}$ 3	M	20
5.	Back Squat	$\frac{50}{5}$ $\frac{55}{5}$ $\frac{60}{5}$ 4	S	30
6.	Bench Press	$\frac{55}{5}$ $\frac{65}{4}$ $\frac{75}{4}$ 3	M	21
7.	Chin-ups			
8.	Plyometrics - Hayes Hops			
	1. Double on Top	3 series x 8 platforms		
	2. Double in Hole	" "		
	3. Single on Top	" "		
	4. Single in Hole	" "		
9.	Ballistics - Standing Drills			
	1. Two Hand Chest Throw	3 sets x 8 reps		
	2. Standing Overhead Throw	" "		
10.	Weighted Sit-ups	$\frac{25 \text{ lbs.}}{10}$ 3		
*	Relaxation and Flexibility			
	1. Chin-up Pull Downs	3 x 8 seconds		
	2. Side to Side	3 x 6 reps		
	3. Split Squat Stretch	3 x 5 reps		

Total Reps __139__

Personal Training Record

Date: Friday - example   Time: _____   _____ Training

Body weight before training _____   After it _____

Self-feeling before training _____

During the time of training _____

After training _____

Notions of the coach _____

Number of exercises in order	Name of exercise	Volume and intensity	Zone S = Small M = Medium B = Big	Total number of Repetitions
✻	Warm-up Routine			
	1. One-legged Squat	3 sets × 6 reps		
	2. Glute Ham Raises	3 sets × 8 reps		
	3. Shoulder Flexers	3 sets × 10 reps		
	4. Standing Long Jumps	1 set × 9 reps		
1.	Snatch Pull	$\frac{50}{4}$ 2 $\frac{60}{4}$ 4	S	24
2.	Split Snatch	$\frac{50}{4}$ $\frac{55}{3}$ $\frac{60}{4}$ 2 $\frac{65}{3}$ $\frac{70}{3}$ 2	M	24
3.	Clean and Jerk	$\frac{50}{3}$ $\frac{60}{3}$ 2 $\frac{70}{4}$ 3	M	21
4.	Front Squat	$\frac{55}{4}$ $\frac{65}{3}$ 3 $\frac{75}{3}$ $\frac{85}{2}$ 3	B	22
5.	Closed Grip Bench Press	$\frac{55}{4}$ $\frac{65}{4}$ 2 $\frac{75}{4}$ $\frac{80}{3}$ 3	B	25
6.	Dips	$\frac{25 lbs}{6}$ 4		
7.	Plyometrics - Speed - Strength Running Drills			
	1. Skips	60 yards × 4 reps		
	2. Bounds	" " " "		
	3. Running A's	" " " "		
8.	Ballistics - Floor Drills			
	1. Kneeling Overhead Throw	3 sets × 8 reps		
	2. Sit-up Throw	" " " "		
9.	Weighted Sit-ups	$\frac{25 lbs}{10}$ 3		
✻	Relaxation and Flexibility			
	1. Chin-up Pull Downs	3 × 8 seconds		
	2. Side to Side	3 × 6 reps		
	3. Split Squat Stretch	3 × 5 reps		

Total Reps ___116___

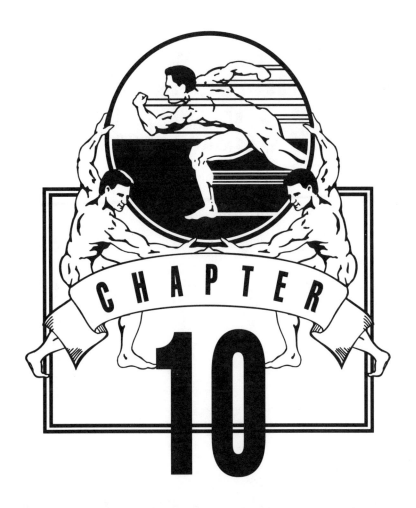

CHAPTER 10

MOTIVATIONAL TECHNIQUES IN SPEED-STRENGTH TRAINING

"In front of excellence, the immortal gods have put sweat, and long and steep is the way to it."
Hesiod
Philosopher

MOTIVATIONAL TECHNIQUES IN SPEED-STRENGTH TRAINING

To teach an athlete how to sustain his motivation, the coach may want to incorporate the use of the following steps in the speed-strength training program:

1. Set short-term goals--not just in football, but in school, work and speed-strength training.

2. Setting long-term goals may lead to long-range results; work with the athlete for what is and what could be down the road.

3. Help the athletes learn about the major motivating forces in their lives.

4. Establish a schedule--the success of any program depends on the players having a well-planned day-to-day, as well as a month-to-month, program with goals and objectives.

5. Teach that anything worth working for has a price to be paid; it is just who wants it the most. Key on the end result. Make pain a positive factor.

6. Teach what all-out effort is--and the enjoyment of the sensation that comes from achieving this effort.

7. Teach the players to understand the challenge in preparing--by learning more and more; reconstruct and construct new speed-strength training regimens as their knowledge of training develops.

8. Learn to enjoy success.

9. Motivate players to success; success is what you and the coach say it is. Success depends upon the goals of each player and the follow-through.

10. Teach by example--the coach who is enthusiastic and excited about his team always has a better chance of success.

TRAINER AND COACH AS A MOTIVATOR

The trainer and coach should be a motivator. One task of the coach involved in a speed-strength program is to consistently motivate his athletes to higher and higher levels. The following principles apply to the coach in using motivational principles that encourage participation of the football player:

1. The coach must motivate the players to get involved in speed-strength training at the very beginning; then he should keep encouraging them over the sticking points--those dead periods when strength gains and speed gains come slowly.

2. By being there to help and support, the football coach can promote this new confidence and build from what the athlete sees changing in his own body. He sees the strength and speed improve in the form of greater strength and body mass, and he sees himself getting better. Doyle Kenady, Coach of the 1983 United States Powerlifting Team, says that to enjoy success "in any sport, an athlete has to have a lot of drive and motivation. Talent isn't enough. *Everybody at the top level has talent.*"

Often at the beginning of training, the coach must downplay the thinking that "if some is good, then more is better" philosophy of training. The coach/trainer should be there on hand for every workout, especially in the beginning weeks of any phase.

3. The coach should know that not all athletes respond to the same type of motivational techniques.

PROMOTING SPEED-STRENGTH TRAINING

The coach who plans, formulates and executes a speed-strength training program designed to build a stronger and faster football team understands that this means he must improve the levels of all of his players, and not just concentrate on a select few.

The following are some motivating methods that have been used in inspiring football players to better themselves.

PHOTOGRAPHS

One coach takes Polaroid snapshots of early beginning stages of his athletes and then takes periodical shots every so often so that the players can see the progress made. Posting photographs of individual team members who are working out using different exercises and movements on the bulletin board in the weight room is an added incentive to train hard.

RECORD BOARDS

This is an excellent way of encouraging the players to compete against others, as well as themselves. Being recognized as one of "the best" is a motivating reward and will hopefully encourage others to follow. Record boards also can break down not only team records, but also personal records that can motivate all the team members to work to excel.

MONTHLY PROGRESS REPORTS

Monthly progress reports help remind each team member about his goals and his progress thus far. Also, they let the athletes know that the coach is overseeing their work--good or bad.

TESTING

The testing days should be at the end of each cycle. It will help the athletes if they are taught and coached how to prepare for a testing session. *The coach can use the testing period the same as he would use the game preparation day--teaching how to be confident and ready to succeed without fear of failure.*

TEAM CONTEST

Outside of the testing days, the use of team contests is excellent for peaking out of testing periods and also allows the coach to use rewards in the form of T-shirts, trophies, medals and other school athletic wear. T-shirts can promote the school nickname or team motto as a reward for a certain level met or proficiency in a particular movement. Trophies and medals can be used in the team contest to reward the best performance. Also, these events provide an opportunity to invite parents, friends, fans and local junior athletes to come and watch.

MOTTOS AND QUOTAS

The use of mottos, slogans and quotas in the weight room and/or in the dressing room is another excellent motivation technique. To further instill pride in the weight room itself can be a great motivating factor for all team members. A well-kept, clean and spirited training facility can make the difference in how athletes interpret the seriousness of the coach. It is amazing what a little paint and cleaning can do. It is not uncommon for parents to become concerned with and involved in helping refurbish or create a better training site for their sons. *Again, a little enthusiasm and will power can go a long way in teaching young men how to win.*

SPECIAL AWARDS

The football coach who does keep up-to-date, accurate records of the progress of his football team can yearly select the outstanding individuals who complement the speed-strength training program and acknowledge their accomplishment. The incorporation of special awards, medals, trophies or certificates to accompany these achievements works as a positive motivating factor for all team members to become more totally involved and dedicated. Special athletic wear (T-shirts, shorts, hats and sweats) can serve the place of trophies as incentive gifts. The pride that is exemplified by the recipient of such a special award sets an example for others to follow. The special awards allow the football coach an opportunity to identify the not-so-talented players who are participating and working to help the team achieve its goals.

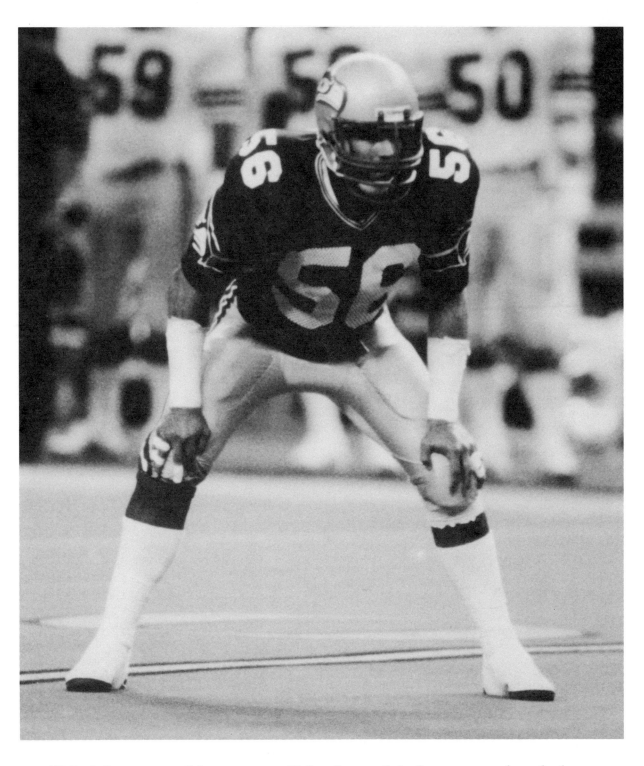

"Hold yourself responsible for a higher standard than anybody else expects of you."
Henry Ward Beecher
Minister

GLOSSARY

Listed on the following pages are some of the main terms of vocabulary in speed-strength training. Throughout the book, the terminology plays an important role in understanding concepts, basic terms and accepted definitions of speed-strength training.

Absolute strength	maximum amount of weight lifted, regardless of the amount of time
Acceleration sprints	a type of sprint training characterized by a building up to full speed, then gradually slowing down, and repeating again
Active rest	period of time off from regular training routine, includes activities of a different nature
Aerobic exercise	exercise which utilizes oxygen
Agility	the ability to change direction rapidly, while maintaining balance (without the loss of speed)
Agonist	a contracting muscle or group of muscles
Anaerobic exercise	high-intensity exercise that exceeds the body's aerobic capacity and builds up an oxygen debt. (Because of its high intensity, anaerobic exercise can be continued for only a short time. A typical anaerobic exercise would be full-speed sprinting on a track.)
Antagonist	the muscle on the opposite side of the joint from where the muscles are being worked. (For example, if working on the biceps, the triceps are the antagonist; if working on the triceps, the biceps are the antagonist.)
Arm-pull	too energetic inclusion into work of one or both arms in performing the snatch or jerk, following a slowing down or a pause
Average weight in training	relation of total sum of weight lifted in training in good style to the number of lifts of the bar
Balance	the ability to control the body's position, whether stationary (as in a hand stand) or moving (as in gymnastics stunts)
Balanced program	a conditioning program that develops the overall body, working each muscle group properly
Ballistics	the throwing of over-weighted or under-weighted objects using different increments of weights
Bar	the iron or steel shaft that forms the handle of a barbell or dumbbell (Barbell bars vary in length from about four to seven feet, while dumbbell bars are twelve to sixteen inches long. Bars are usually one inch in diameter and are often cased in a revolving sleeve.)

Barbell	This is the basic piece of equipment for weight training (It consists of a bar, sleeve, collars and plates. The weight of an adjustable barbell without plates averages five pounds per foot of bar length. The weight of this basic barbell unit must be required training poundage. These poundages are designated by numerals painted or engraved on the sides of the plates.)
Barbell curl	performed by raising the barbell in an underhand contraction of the bicep muscles of the arms
Basic movement skills	skills that can be performed at an early age -- such as jumping, catching and climbing to improve coordination
Basic training weight	weight of the bar with which the athlete normally trains
Bench press	one of the lifting events contested in powerlifting competition (The exercise is instituted by lowering the barbell downward to the chest and then raising it from the chest to an upward position. The athlete's position is in a supine, lying position on the lifting bench.)
Biathlon	the classical lifts performed under complex and definite rules
Body builder	a person who develops the physique through a combination of exercises and diet for the purpose of competition and exhibition
Body building	a subdivision of the general category of weight training in which the main objective is to change the appearance of the human body via heavy weight training and applied nutrition
Body composition	the ratio of lean body mass to body fat
Cheating	a method of swinging the weights or body to complete a repetition that would have otherwise been impossible
Classical lifts	lifts which make up the program of competitions in weight lifting, e.g., consisting of the snatch and clean jerk
Clean	the act of raising a barbell or dumbbell to shoulder height
Clean and jerk	classical lift in which the bar is lifted to the chest in one movement and then jerked to arms' length overhead in a second movement
Close spot	to be alert and ready to assist when called upon by someone performing an exercise
Collar	on barbells, a clamp that secures the plate on the bar
Competitive phase	phase of training that takes place during the competitive period or season
Contraction	the shortening of the length of a muscle

Coordination	the combination of power, agility, balance, skill, flexibility and endurance of the athletic movement
Dead lift	one of the lifting events contested in powerlifting competition (The exercise is instituted by positioning the athlete against the barbell on the floor. The legs are then bent. One hand is palm down and the other palm is up. The athlete pulls the barbell from the floor until standing in an erect position.)
Dexterity	athlete agility, balance and coordination
Distortion	lag of the flexing of one arm during the lifting of the bar
Drop	executed after the barbell is pulled in an upward movement, as in the clean and snatch exercises where the athlete is to move under the moving weight
Dumbbell	A shorter version of a barbell, which is intended for use in one hand or, more commonly, with equally weighted dumbbells in each hand (All of the characteristics and terminology of a barbell are the same in a dumbbell.)
Dynamic start	a start with a preparatory movement in order to develop inertial movement of the body and strength of reaction while on the feet
Easy set	to describe the performance of an exercise indicating it was not close to maximum effort
Elite athletes	considered the very best in athletics sports, the highest degree of ranking one can have
Exercise	(Used as a noun, this is the actual speed-strength movement executed (e.g., a bench press or power clean). An exercise is often called a movement. Used as a verb, to exercise is to work out physically and recreationally with weight training or any number of other forms of exercise.)
Explosive strength	maximum amount of force exerted in a certain extension period of time
Extension	the return of any joint to the anatomical position
Fixation	holding the bar overhead at arms' length in conformity to competition rules
Flex	to bend or curve the arm, to contract or extend a muscle
Flexibility	the ability to flex and extend the joints through their fully intended range of motion without being impeded by excessive tissue (fat or muscle) or tightness in tissue (connective tissue or muscle)
Force	the capacity for exerting strength

Forced reps	a method of training whereby a training partner helps lift a weight just enough so the movement can be completed for two or three repetitions once the trainee has reached a point where he cannot complete it on his own
Free hand exercise	exercise that can be performed without equipment, using body weight for the resistance of one muscle group against another
Full extension	maximum effort in the pull above the level of the knees
Full range-of-motion	the greatest range possible for a muscle or group of muscles
Functional overload	a change in the resistance that is normally used to help stimulate the explosive starting and absolute strength needed to surpass the goal or standard (Medicine balls, weighted implements and weighted objects—shot put, discus and hammer are examples.)
Gear	training clothes and equipment used for athletic endeavors
Grip	method of gripping the bar in the hands
Grip width	width between the hands on the knurling of the bar
Half-squat	drop while bending the legs only slightly at the knees
Hand off	assisting in getting a weight in proper position to commence an exercise
Hard set	description used to indicate a near maximum effort used to perform a prescribed number of repetitions of an exercise
Hook grip	grip where the thumb is covered by the middle fingers
Hyperextension	extension of a limb to a greater degree than the normal maximal extension
In-season program	a program to be used while competing to maintain the strength and conditioning levels that have been achieved by the preseason program
Intensity	the amount of weight lifted
Interval sprints	a type of sprint training characterized by sprinting at full speed, followed by a specified recovery time, then repeating
Jerk	second part of the clean and jerk (Movement starts from the chest and is continued overhead.)
Kilograms	part of the metric system of weight and mass (One kilo equals 2.2046 pounds, or 1,000 grams.)
Knee-bend	movement of knees forward during the lift
Knee-touch	touching the platform with the knee when lowering the body under the bar in the split

Knurling	coarse part or section of a barbell or dumbbell where the grip of hands is placed
Lean body mass	lean body weight minus body fat
Leg thrust	help from the thighs during lifting
Lift from the hang	lifting the bar, which is held in the hands at waist height
Lift off	assisting in getting a weight in proper position to commence an exercise
Lifting belt	a leather or nylon belt four to six inches wide at the back that is worn around the waist to protect a trainee's lower back and abdomen from injuries (The six-inch belt can be used in training, but only the four-inch belt can be used in actual weight-lifting competition.)
Lifting platform	a designated section built to support performance of weight-lifting exercises -- a designated area with limits and boundaries
Load	amount of weight
Lock-out	executing a partial repetition of an exercise by pushing a weight through the last few inches of the movement
Major exercise	an exercise that directly improves one's athletic performance
Master of sport	highest degree of ranking in athletic supremacy in the Soviet Union
Motivation	anything that impels a person to keep moving toward a goal
Muscular endurance	the ability to withstand isolated and overall effects of fatigue on the body during prolonged work
Non-locks	performing an exercise without moving the weight through the complete range of motion at the top failing to lock out the elbows or knees
Odd lifts	exercises other than the snatch and clean and jerk which are used for competition such as the squat, bench press or barbell curl
Off-season program	a program to be used while not competing to enhance strength and conditioning levels
Olympic barbell	a highly specialized and finely machined barbell used in weight-lifting competition and heavy bodybuilding training (An Olympic barbell weighs 20 kilograms (slightly less than forty-five pounds), and each of its collars weighs 2 1/2 kilograms (5.5 pounds.)
Olympic lifting	a form of competitive weight lifting included in the Olympic Games program since the revival of the modern Olympics at Athens in 1896 (Until 1972, this form of weight lifting consisted of three lifts: the press, snatch and clean and jerk. Because of officiating difficulties, however, the press was dropped from use following the 1972 Olympic Games,

	leaving the snatch and clean and jerk as the two competitive Olympic lifts.)
Olympic plates	weights that have a two-inch diameter center hole, for use with an Olympic bar
Olympic set	a weight set that includes a seven-foot, two-inch revolving bar, and plates that have a two-inch diameter hole
One-hundred-ten-pound set	a standard bar with locks, in addition to an assortment of 10, 5, 2 1/2 and 1 1/2 pound standard plates that total 110 pounds
Opening out	straightening of the trunk and legs after the effort to achieve full extension
Opposite grip	grip where the palms face in opposite directions
Overhand grip	grip where the palms face backwards
Overload	a degree of stress placed on the muscle that is over and above the amount the muscle is ordinarily used to handling
Overtraining	a state of reduced muscle size and strength which occurs as a result of working at too high an intensity, or not allowing enough recovery time over a long period of time
Partial reps	performing an exercise without moving the weight through the complete range of motion at either the beginning of a repetition or at the end of the repetition, not making a complete contraction or extension of the muscle
Pause	short halting of the movement of the bar
Peak athletic performance	when all the elements of training display themselves at the highest level of competition, thus elevating the essence of performance to the best the athlete has to offer at this moment in time
Periodization	annual plan that is divided into training phases
Plyometrics	revolves around jump activities involving explosiveness, generated force in the shortest amount of time
Power lifting	a competitive situation in which individuals try to lift as much as possible for one repetition, each on three exercises: squat, bench press and deadlift
Preparatory phase	phase of training that leads into a precompetitive competition or preseason
Pressing grip	width of grip suitable for executing the press
Pull	lifting of the bar from the platform to the "drop"

Pull with drop	pull executed without bending the legs after the full extension
Reaction strength	speed in which the initial body movement causes an opposite and increased movement from the second movement that occurs to the follow-through
Recovery	standing of the athlete into upright position with the bar on the chest or arms' length overhead after a lift
Recovery time	the time necessary for the muscles to rebuild themselves after being torn down during a workout
Repetitions	number of attempts that make up a set
Rest between sets	the amount of time taken between the conclusion of one set and the beginning of the next set
Rest intervals	duration of rest between workouts
Sets	series of repetitions in a given order
Simple grip	grip in which the four fingers are on the side, the thumb on the other side of the bar
Single rhythm lift	lift of bar to the drop with emphasis on effort at moment of full extension
Snatch	classical lift in which the bar is lifted overhead onto straight arms in one movement
Snatch grip	width of grip suitable for executing the snatch
Speed	the distance covered per unit of time
Speed-strength	the combination of maximum speed incorporated in maximum strength, thus producing the greatest amount of power (There are four components of speed-strength: absolute, explosive, starting and reaction.)
Split drop	drop while bending the legs, one forward, one straight back
Spotter	person who aids the lifter
Squat	one of the lifting events contested in power-lifting competition (The exercise is instituted by positioning the athlete standing under the barbell with the weight balanced on his shoulders and back. Then he performs a deep knee bend of lowering the body with the weight on the shoulders and back until the tops of the thighs are below parallel.)
Squat drop	drop while bending the legs, with feet placed to either side
Standard bar	a solid one-inch bar, either five or six feet in length

Standard plates	weights that have a 1 1/8-inch diameter hole for use with a standard bar
Start	initial position for lifting the bar from the platform
Starting strength	measure of how fast and forceful the movement is at its beginning
Starting weight	weight with which the athlete begins his first attempt in a contest
Static start	motionless pose from which the athlete lifts the bar
Sticking point	any point of a movement that is very difficult to get past in order to complete the movement
Strength	the degree of ability to apply or resist force
Strength training	a type of training that involves an increase in strength to enhance athletic performance
Stretching	a type of exercise program used to promote body flexibility (It involves assuming and then holding postures in which certain muscle groups and body joints are stretched.)
Stride frequency	number of strides taken per second
Stride length	the distance covered in one stride
Supplementary exercise	an exercise that indirectly improves athletic performance
Techniques	the proper method of performance for an exercise or drill
Thumbless grip	grip where all fingers and the thumb are on one side of the bar
Training cycle	phases of periodization dealing with the amount of volume and intensity
Training goals	the desired performance levels an athlete is working toward
Training load	the poundage used for workouts
Training plateau	state attained when strength gains peak and levels off
Training to failure	method of training whereby the trainee has continued to set a point where it is impossible for him to complete another rep without assistance
Transition phase	phase of time that follows the preparatory periods and competitive periods, time of active rest
Twist	turning of trunk and bar to one side during lifting
Underhand grip	grip where the palms face forward

Volume	the number of repetitions completed in a set
Volume of load	total weight lifted in training
Warm-up weight	weight with which the athlete limbers up before lifting weights
Weight	another term for <u>poundage</u> or <u>resistance</u> (Sometimes this term is used generally to refer to the apparatus (barbell, dumbbell etc.) being used in an exercise, versus the exact poundage being used in an exercise.)
Weight lifting	the subdivision of weight training in which men and women compete in weight classes both nationally and internationally to see who can lift the heaviest weights for single repetitions in prescribed exercises
Weight training	a type of training that results in increased strength for improvement in fitness
Wraps	pieces of material to wrap certain joints of the body for additional support

REFERENCES

Bennett, J. C., & Pravitz, J. E. (1982). *The miracle of sports psychology*. Englewood Cliffs, NJ: Prentice-Hall.

Bompa, T. 0. (1983). *Theory and methodology of training - the key to athletic performance*. Dubuque, IA: Kendall/Hunt

Costello, F. (1984). *Bounding to the top—the complete book on plyometric training*. College Park, MD: University of Maryland.

Dintiman, G. (1984). *How to run faster—step-by-step by-step instruction on how to increase foot speed*. West Point, NY: Leisure Press.

Dobbins, B. (1985, January). How much is too much. *Sports Fitness*, 71-73, 115.

Ferguson, H. E. (1982). *The edge*. Fairview Park, OH: Author.

Fixx, J. F. (1985). *Maximum sports performance*. New York: Random House.

Goldstein, G. (1988, December). Seminar on speed-strength training, East Rutherford, NJ.

Harris, H. A. (1966). *Greek athletes and athletics*. Bloomington, IN: Indiana University Press.

Hatfield, F. C. (1985, April). Power and the legs. *Sports Fitness*, 87-89, 116.

Jesse, J. P. (1978). Misuse of strength development programs. *National Strength Coaches Association* Journal, 2(1), 18-20.

Medvedev, A. S., Rodionov, V. I., Rogozyan, V. N., & Melkonyan, A. A. (1979). Periodization of weightlifting training. Soviet Sports Review, 14(4), 196201.

Murray, A., & Lear, J. (1981). *Power training for sport*. New York: Arco.

O'Shea, P. (1985, August). Throwing speed. *Sports Fitness*, 66-69, 89-90.

Pedersen, G. (1985, April). Technologies of power. *Sports Fitness*, 84-85, 119.

Raiport, G. (1988). *"Red gold"—Peak performance techniques of the Russian and East German Olympic Victor*. Los Angeles, CA: Jeremy P. Tarcher.

Roy, A., & Gillman, S. (1964). *World champion San Diego Chargers strength program—in and out of season*. San Diego: Author.

Starr, B. (1978). *The strongest shall survive*. Washington: D. C.: Fitness Products.

Steinhaus, A. H. (1963). *Training for strength in sports, toward an understanding of health and physical education*. Duguque, IA: William C. Brown.

Sutherland, J. (1988). *Choosing free weight equipment—a design, function and value survey*. Paper presented at the Universal Gym Equipment Sales Meeting and Product Design Seminar, Cedar Rapids, IA.

Swanbom, D. (1977). *Strength of the UCLA Bruins*. Los Angeles: Author

Verhoshansky, Y. (1967, December). Are depth jumps useful? *Track and Field*, 9.

Vorobyev, A. N. (1978). *Weightlifting*. (W. J. Brice, Trans.). Budapest, Hungary: International Weightlifting Federation. Vorbyev, A. N. (1979). The scientific basis of weightlifting training and technique. *Soviet Sports Review* 14(1), 1-5.

Webster, D . (1976) . *The iron game—an illustrated history of weightlifting*. Irvine, Ayrshire, Scotland: Author.

Yessis, M. (1981) . The role of specificity in strength training for track, gymnastics, and other sports. *National Strength and Conditioning Association Journal, 2* (5), 20-21, 47 .

Yessis, M. (1982). Additional thoughts on strength and power. *National Strength and Conditioning Association* Journal, 4(5), 24-25.

Yessis, M. (1983). The role of specialized training in multi-year and yearly training programs. *National* Strength and Conditioning Association Journal, 4(6), 10-11, 36.

Yessis, M. (1984, September). Soviet training concepts-speed-strength training. *Strength and Health*, 20-30.

Yessis, M. (1985, April). The Soviet power machine. *Sports Fitness*, 75-77.

Yessis, M. (1987). *Secrets of Soviet sports fitness and training*. New York: Arbor House.

Yessis, M., & Hatfield, F. C. (1986). *Plyometric* training—achieving explosive power in sports. Canoga Park, CA: Fitness Systems.

NOTES

NOTES